GOAL DIGGER FITNESS

Look, Feel, and Perform Your Best with a Breakthrough 14-Day Exercise Plan

Eric Harr

WITH **ALEXA JOY SHERMAN**

RODALE

NOTICE

The information in this book is meant to supplement, not replace, proper exercise training.
All forms of exercise pose some inherent risks. The editors and publisher advise readers
to take full responsibility for their safety and know their limits. Before practicing the exercises
in this book, be sure that your equipment is well maintained, and do not take risks beyond
your level of experience, aptitude, training, and fitness. The exercise and dietary programs
in this book are not intended as a substitute for any exercise routine or dietary regimen
that may have been prescribed by your doctor. As with all exercise and dietary programs,
you should get your doctor's approval before beginning.

Mention of specific companies, organizations, or authorities in this book does not imply
endorsement by the publisher, nor does mention of specific companies,
organizations, or authorities imply that they endorse this book.

Internet addresses and telephone numbers given in this book were accurate
at the time it went to press.

Rodale books may be purchased for business or promotional use or
for special sales. For information, please write to:

Special Markets Department, Rodale Inc., 733 Third Avenue, New York, NY 10017

Printed in the United States of America

Rodale Inc. makes every effort to use acid-free ∞, recycled paper ♻.

Photographs by Tom MacDonald

Book design by Susan Eugster

Library of Congress Cataloging-in-Publication Data

Harr, Eric, date
     Goal digger fitness : look, feel, and perform your best with a breakthrough 14-day exercise
plan / Eric Harr with Alexa Joy Sherman.
         p.   cm.
     Includes index.
     ISBN 13 978–1–59486–438–4   paperback
     ISBN 10 1–59486–438–1   paperback
     1. Physical fitness—Handbooks, manuals, etc.   2. Exercise—Handbooks, manuals, etc.
I. Sherman, Alexa Joy.   II. Title.
GV481.H2554   2007
613.7—dc22   2007008414

Distributed to the trade by Holtzbrinck Publishers

2   4   6   8   10   9   7   5   3   1   hardcover

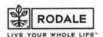

We inspire and enable people to improve their lives and the world around them

For more of our products visit rodalestore.com or call 800-848-4735

Contents

Acknowledgments

Each time I sit down to write the acknowledgments for a book, I get a little self-conscious because I feel like I'm crafting a sappy, cheesy acceptance speech ("... you love me, you reeeeally love me!"). But the simple fact is that acknowledgments are important—they allow me to sappily and cheesily recognize the people who genuinely help make a project not just possible but better and more meaningful than it would have been if I'd gone it alone.

That said, there are dozens of people who matter to me and who, in some way, have supported me and have helped me do what I do. For this book, however, I'll keep my list of acknowledgments to three lovely ladies:

Alexa Joy Sherman. You are such a sweet woman—and a talented writer. Thank you for taking on a project you knew would be trouble (!)—and for baking so much love, emotion, and humor into these pages.

My remarkable wife, Alexandra. For those of you who don't know, I met Alex (I call her Brandy; that's her middle name) when I was 17 years old. And today, 18 years later, our relationship remains as warm and fuzzy and

< v >

new and magical as when we met. I have you to thank for that, Brandy. You work so hard at our relationship. You are the most soulful, loving, and unflinchingly loyal person I have ever known—and the idea that we have created my next, and final, acknowledgment together always fills my heart with immeasurable gratitude.

And now to you, my dear Vivienne. At 2½ years old, you're not quite old enough to read these words—but at the rate you are learning (way faster than most kids, of course!), you will soon enough be able to read this. So, here's the thing: I always thought that love was finite; that you could only love someone so much; that the human heart, a cardiac muscle roughly the size of one's fist, had tangible limits on how much love it could pour out. You, my sweet, have proven that notion categorically wrong. Every night when I kiss your velvety head as you drift off to dream, I think to myself: "I couldn't love this little person any more than I do." Then, the next morning when you jolt me out of sleep by clambering onto my bed, hollering "Papaaa!" I look into your smiling eyes, and I realize I had more love in there after all. This cycle has repeated itself so many times I've conceded that love is, indeed, infinitely deep and infinitely powerful. And you've taught this to me simply by being you. Thank you, Viv, for teaching me life's most precious lesson. I love you infinity-infinity (plus one ... every morning!).

Introduction
The "Goal Digger" in You

No doubt you've heard about the obesity epidemic in America. And when you take in the startling stats, you probably think, "Thank goodness I'm not a part of *that* societal scourge." No, not you. You've been active your whole life—at least, you've tried to be.

Even now, with everything you've got going on, from work to family to social obligations, you're able to squeeze in a workout here and there, to hit the weight room or the yoga mat or a Spinning or Pilates or Fusion Booty Ballet class; to play a game of hoops with your buddies on the weekend; or to walk with your neighbor once or twice a week. Or perhaps you consider yourself a runner, cyclist, beach volleyballer, golfer, or Rollerblader. Then again, maybe you're at the point where you just take the stairs instead of the elevator, do some yard work or vacuum the living room vigorously, park in the farthest spot from the entrance when you shop, and talk to your coworkers instead of e-mailing them (hey, all the fitness magazines say these things

< **vii** >

count as calorie-burning activities!). Whatever the case, you lead a reasonably active life—when you have the time and, of course, motivation. Bottom line: You're not a member of the lethargic class of couch potatoes that just can't seem to find anything appealing about exercise. You like to move, and you do so whenever you can (and whenever life allows!).

But lately, "whenever you can," and "whenever life allows," may not be as often as you'd like it to be—certainly not as often as it used to be. Do a little soul-searching and be honest with yourself: When was the last time you *really* exercised at your optimum target heart rate (between 60 and 90 percent of your maximum, according to the American College of Sports Medicine)? How long has it been since you logged regular, consistent workouts on a weekly or monthly—never mind yearly—basis? If you're like most people, it's been too long. In fact, studies indicate less than half of all adults who participate in some form of physical activity actually engage in it frequently or intensely enough to reap any significant health benefits.

Which brings me to another point (and I don't mean to come on so strong, so early in our relationship, but this is important stuff!): Perhaps it's not just that you haven't found the time to be consistently active but that you're not entirely sure how to get the most out of the exercise you *do* get. Sure, you may know your way around a set of dumbbells, but are you doing the right moves for your body and skill level, using the optimum amount of weight, mixing things up enough, giving yourself sufficient rest and recovery time? Or perhaps you love a good game of tennis but find said game remains consistently at the same level. Maybe you've been practicing yoga for months, even years, but your body has stayed in the same sort of shape almost as long. Then there's that cardio program you've been doing your whole life: same settings on the same machine or the same RPE on the same route, day in, day out, *ad nauseum!* But do you even know what RPE means, or that your body likely adapted to your workout a long time ago?

I'm not trying to criticize here but merely to point out that most people who exercise or play a sport or do anything remotely active often lack the information needed to excel in those activities (yes, even I was in the dark about how to succeed as a triathlete back when I first started), and just as many don't devote nearly as much time to their fitness as they'd like to (or should). They are the "moderately active" masses, neither sedentarily obese nor supremely fit. But those people—like you—*want* to kick their training up a notch (or even several notches, depending upon the starting point). They *want* to be able to strike the word *moderately* from their fitness profile and simply be active, perhaps even "hyper" active, if such a term didn't mean "child in need of Ritalin."

There is in each of us a fitness goal digger, a person who thrives upon movement, who is ready to set exercise goals and do what it takes to achieve them. In fact, even sedentary couch potatoes have an active little nugget deep down—the kid who used to chase a ball with his friends, to ride her bike over hills and along sidewalks, to breathlessly wait for recess to begin, hula-hooping and hopscotching and wishing the days were longer so she could jump rope just a few more minutes ("Mom, pleeease!"). Unfortunately, we all grew up. Now, being active is probably just one more thing you have to squeeze into your daily schedule. It may still be something you enjoy when you get a chance to do it, but you've lost sight of how to make it work within the context of your day-to-day life. Whether you're that former playful child who matured too quickly; an ex-college runner who has fallen out of shape while working too much; a busy mom who needs practical strategies to integrate fitness into family life; or the person who simply needs a fresh, motivating fitness program—*you* are a goal digger. I'm going to show you how to access and unleash that person once more.

It's time to start playing again and to feel truly alive, vital, and your fittest ever. I may not even need to motivate you to move but, rather, to simply show you how to move a bit harder or faster or more frequently than you have been. Either way, it's going to be easier—and a whole lot more enjoyable—than you might think.

The way I see it, taking your fitness to the next level can be achieved in three relatively simple steps. First, you'll evaluate what's been holding you back all this time, keeping you in something of a healthy-body holding pattern—if not a decline. Second, you will define in no uncertain terms what you want from the activities you perform—no more nebulous wishes for a "better" body or "improved" performance; those will be the big-picture goals, to be sure, but then you're going to get intensely specific, so there's no wiggle room. Third, you'll get rolling with a 14-Day Program that not only takes those specific goals into account, but also considers your daily schedule, energy levels, and physical abilities—and that's fantastically *fun*. The beauty of this third step lies in the entirely doable (and easily digestible!)

14-Day Programs I've mapped out to help you reach your goals, all while taking your psychology, physiology, and available time into account. Thrown in along the way are a slew of strategies to keep your fires stoked—from ways to sculpt your mind as you strengthen your body to skill-building, injury-preventing advice to power-eating plans.

Now, is taking your fitness to the next level already sounding seriously simple? That's the spirit! It is.

Let's get moving.

GOAL
DIGGER
FITNESS

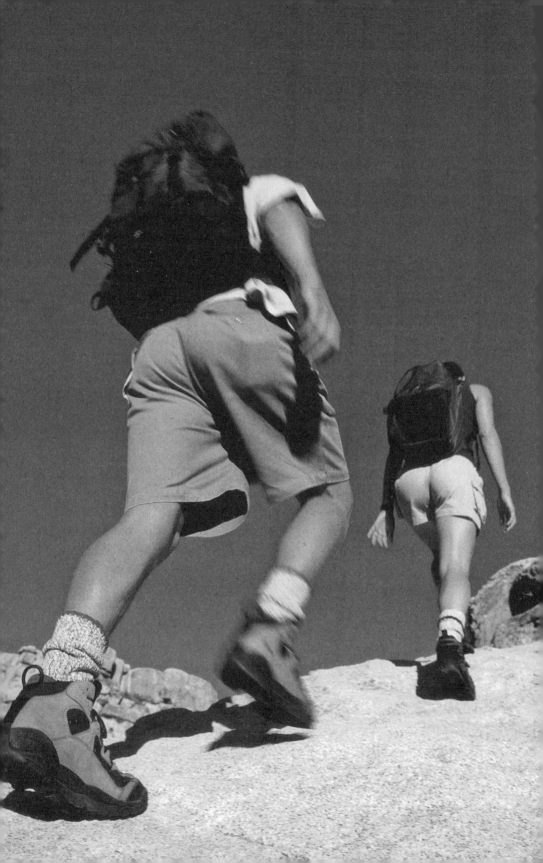

ONE

Get Over It: Pushing Past Roadblocks in Your Quest for Greater Fitness

"Success consists of getting up just one more time than you fall."
—English author Oliver Goldsmith

Okay, I'm going to give it to you straight: If you've lost sight of how much you love being active, you've stopped pushing your body and have consequently deprived yourself of the ability to see just how magnificently it can perform, or you've been taking your passion to move—on any level—for granted, well, you've allowed something to get in your way. Yes, I'm suggesting *you* let that happen. I know this will sound like psychobabble or some trite form of self-help jargon, but only in taking responsibility for whatever roadblocks or snags are stopping you can you reclaim the power and push past them. In fact, when you take control, you'll likely realize these issues, obstacles, barriers, excuses—whatever you want to call them—are not

< 1 >

nearly as insurmountable as they've seemed up until now. After all, you probably got over similar hurdles (or didn't even know—or pretend—they existed) way back when you were performing at your peak, even if that time was during a game of tag when you were 5.

So before you put a plan in motion—before you even *think* about what you want to achieve and why—you've got to identify and resolve what's been holding you back, physically and/or mentally, up until now. If you don't

goaldigger*inspiration*

Working Mom Gets Better Body, Improves Health

Julie Russell, 40, a mother of two and a third-grade teacher from Riverside, California, went from walking on a treadmill a couple times a week to a powered-up regimen of kickboxing, running, and cycling. What prompted this incredible transformation? "I realized that my age and activity level weren't working together like they used to," Russell says. "The moderate activity didn't bring about results like it did in my 20s." Of course, like anyone, Russell faced challenges: "I have a busy schedule. My kids are 11 and 14, and I work full-time, so there is plenty of homework, chores, et cetera, and little 'extra' time for exercise." How does she do it, then? "I work out where and when the kids do karate. That guarantees me three workouts a week," she says. "I can also leave them at home for an hour now if I want to work out when they don't—and I fixed up our bikes so we can ride together on the weekends."

The payoffs for Russell are many, including more time with her family (not less!), greater confidence and health, being a role model to her kids and students—and better-fitting clothes. "Confidence is the biggest benefit, but an overall attitude of health and making diet and exercise a priority has permeated our family," Russell says. Her message to you: "In a high-stress world where two-thirds of our country is obese and many people suffer from illnesses that could be prevented, take your health into your own hands. Be the healthiest you can be. You will feel better and look better, and others will follow your lead."

begin by clearing the way for success, it's only a matter of time before you give up.

The good news is you're not alone. Not by a long shot. Everybody faces challenges when it comes to getting into better shape. I certainly had plenty of reasons I believed I couldn't take the leap and train for my first triathlon: I felt too fat and inexperienced (wait, I really *was* too fat and inexperienced!), I owned a bike that was the wrong size for my frame, I had blisters from running, and I just lacked motivation. (Fortunately, I allowed the athlete in me to win out over the self-imposed doubts and fears that would have otherwise stopped me from completing my first multisport—and subsequently traveling the world for a decade as a pretty decent pro triathlete.)

Not only are there plenty of possible obstacles, but they tend to shift over time. One week you're feeling motivated to exercise, but you don't have the time. The next week you have the time, but you don't have the energy. When you finally have the energy *and* the time, you suddenly realize you're at a loss for what to do or where you could possibly do it. These are the stories you tell yourself as you hit the snooze button in the morning, bury yourself in a pile of work on your lunch hour, or head straight home after a long day to catch the latest celebrity gossip on *Entertainment Tonight*.

Here's what I've learned through my own self-searching: The seemingly paralyzing barriers that stand in the way of your fitness resurrection are figments of your imagination, for the most part. I know you're *really* busy; we all are. But some of us still find the time to exercise (like Julie Russell, page 2). I know there are times when you honestly don't think you have the energy to push yourself, day after day. But the people who feel that way and then get over it feel a hundred times better than before (just ask Emily Renninger, page 10). I know it's tough to think about taking on a cross-training program when you're getting older and your body's not working like it used to. But others in the same boat who have eased back into a sensible, even rehabilitative program realize how rejuvenating exercise can be (witness Jan Talbot, page 136).

So what's your excuse? What's keeping you from pushing yourself further than you even realized you could? I'm sure you can rattle off at least a few of your favorites, but let's begin with a little self-test to help you pinpoint the biggest and ostensibly most challenging hurdles you're facing. Then we'll have some fun blowing holes in each and every one!

THE EXERCISE EXCUSES ASSESMENT TEST

This survey is designed to find out what prevents you from truly becoming your all-time fittest self. Here's how it works: You'll be assigned a point value for each statement, depending upon how strongly it resonates with you.

- Place a 0 next to each statement that doesn't sound remotely like it came from you.
- Place a 1 next to each statement that seems like it *might* have come out of your mouth.
- Place a 2 next to each statement that's seriously close to sounding like you—but not quite.
- Place a 3 next to each statement that's so completely you, you're wondering how I got inside your head.

Let's get started!

SECTION ONE

[3] I have a hard time dragging myself out of bed for morning exercise.

[2] Last time I pushed myself in a workout, I felt sore and winded.

[3] Five minutes into my workouts, I want to turn around and head for the couch.

[3] Life used to excite me, but now it just wears me out.

[3] Sooo sleeeepy.

[14] **TOTAL FOR THIS SECTION**

SECTION TWO

[3] Any workout that delivers results requires too much of a time commitment for me.

[2] I try to squeeze in exercise, but there always seems to be something more important vying for my attention.

[3] Between getting ready for work, or making breakfast, or getting the kids off to school, or all of these things and more, who has time for a morning workout?

[0] I'm usually working late or running errands in the evening, so I can't exercise then.

[2] I cancel my plans to exercise almost as frequently as I brush my teeth.

[10] **TOTAL FOR THIS SECTION**

SECTION THREE

[3] Last time I tried to get back in shape, I actually hurt myself.

[0] My body just doesn't work the way it used to.

[3] A challenging workout would probably be more painful than profitable.

[0] I frequently suffer from aches and pains.

[2] I can't get fit again—I'm already too far gone.

[8] **TOTAL FOR THIS SECTION**

SECTION FOUR

[0] I might push myself to exercise harder, but I don't like getting sweaty and smelly.

[1] Exercise just isn't as fun as it used to be.

[3] I prefer cocktails to cardio and desserts to dumbbells.

[0] The gym is for losers, workout videos are ridiculous, and athletics is for Neanderthals.

[0] Are we still talking about exercise? Yawn.

[4] **TOTAL FOR THIS SECTION**

SECTION FIVE

[3] I'm not sure what exercises are best for achieving my fitness goals.

[3] I have yet to see any results from the workouts I've been doing.

[0] I'm not coordinated enough to really break a sweat.

[0] I'm kind of scared to get back in shape.

[2] Today's exercise programs are too complicated (is Yogilates a workout or a coffee drink?).

[8] **TOTAL FOR THIS SECTION**

SECTION SIX

[2] Getting a quality workout would cost too much money.

[3] I don't have the right kind of gear or equipment for *real* exercise.

[3] There are no good classes or workout facilities in my area.

[0] I'm on the road a lot and can't find appropriate places to exercise while traveling.

[2] It's too cold in the winter, too hot in the summer, and too rainy in the spring and fall to exercise.

[10] **TOTAL FOR THIS SECTION**

YOUR RESULTS: If you scored 5 points or more in any section, read the corresponding information that follows.

Section One: You're Tired (And So Are Your Excuses!)

Well, it certainly sounds like your energy is in short supply these days. But I've got some really good news for you: The reason you're feeling so lethargic almost certainly has to do with the fact that you're not exercising often or

The**GoalDigger**Tip

Sleepy? Simply start ... and start simply.

Of course it's tough to put your body in motion when your energy levels are low—so I recommend that when you're feeling lethargic, you just lace up your shoes and start with a five minutes of easy walking or another aerobic activity (which you should do to warm up for any type of exercise anyway). Then, stop and assess how you're feeling—inside and out. This is called the "Five Minute Rule." Is your body revved and ready to go, or are your muscles already feeling fatigued? Are you more alert and waking up, or do you feel like you're going to pass out? If you're genuinely dragging and seriously still exhausted, head home and get back in bed; you're probably in need of some rest and relaxation. But, if I'm guessing correctly, the mere fact that you started moving will get you pumped enough to keep going with the quality workout you determined you were too tired to take on. Oftentimes, our minds tell us we're tired when our bodies are actually eager to go.

hard enough. It may sound counterintuitive, but study after study shows that when you expend energy (with activity), you actually *boost* your energy levels and are better equipped to combat chronic fatigue syndrome.

Meanwhile, exercise releases feel-good, mood-boosting endorphins, so not only will you start looking at workouts in a more positive light, you'll view everything else in life with a slightly sunnier disposition. Yet another bonus: Physical activity helps you sleep better at night (just make sure you don't do anything too intense a few hours before bed), meaning you'll wake more refreshed and pumped up to work out in the morning—and to tackle anything else the day subsequently throws your way. No more rolling over to catch a little more shut-eye, no more dragging groggily and sleepily through your life. Bottom line: Exercise won't deplete your energy supply—it will fuel it.

The**GoalDigger**Tip

If you're crunched for time, exercise early in the day.

You may have a million things going on from the moment you wake up, but your day will probably get even busier as the minutes pass. So set your alarm clock for an hour or even 30 minutes earlier, and squeeze in an exercise session then. Research shows that people who work out in the morning are actually more likely to stick with their exercise long-term than people who plan to be active at other times of day. On top of that, the sense of accomplishment you'll get from the moment your day begins will give you the confidence to conquer even more throughout your day—meaning you could potentially be extra productive on the days you get that a.m. exercise, hence, actually *saving* you time.

Section Two: You're Over-Scheduled (And Under-Exercised)

First, allow me to validate you: People today are absolutely busier than ever, and "lack of time" is the top excuse almost everyone gives for not exercising, hands down. With expenses mounting, families often rely on two incomes to pay the bills, while caring for kids and trying to maintain some semblance of a social life. So yes, it would seem there aren't enough hours in the day to accomplish all these things, let alone to work out. As your daily schedule grows increasingly hectic, exercise gets pushed to the periphery.

However, I think that if you were to examine your time and how you spend it—to really take a good, long look at where each precious minute goes—you'd actually find you have more of it available than you might think. Don't believe me? For the next week, write down exactly what you do from one hour to the next. My guess is you spend 8 or 9 hours a day working and/or taking care of family and the like—and (hopefully) 7 to 9 hours each

The**GoalDigger**Tip

Recruit your relatives.

Are family obligations preventing you from exercising? Then get active with your spouse or partner or kids. It's not only a great way to deal with the "lack of time" excuse but an excellent way to stay motivated while boosting everybody's fitness. Research shows that people who exercise together may stick with it longer than people who go it alone. Besides, what could be more romantic than going on a hike with your significant other, enjoying breathtaking views as you traverse the trails at sunset? And what could be more fun than throwing around a ball with your kids, taking a family bike ride in the park, or heading out with your baby in a jogging stroller?

It's no secret that the obesity epidemic in this country doesn't affect only adults but children as well. And while there are a lot of reasons, I think one of the most compelling is this: These days, kids think of "play" as something that requires a Sony or Nintendo device, and the only sports they enjoy are the ones in which they are virtual athletes on two-dimensional screens. Isn't it time we showed kids it's even cooler to run and jump and skip with their own legs instead of computerized ones? Rope your kids into your workout routine, and everybody benefits.

Meanwhile, studies show that people tend to pack on pounds when they begin a new relationship or get married (something that's become known as the newlywed 9—kind of like the freshman 15, referring to weight college students gain). Why is this? Why does spending time with other people make us less active or entirely inactive? Explore exercise as part of the family experience and see how enriching it is for everyone—mind, body, and soul.

night sleeping (as recommended by the National Sleep Foundation, which also states that Americans typically get 6.9 to 7.5 hours a night). That leaves a good 6 to 9 hours to devote to other things, which may include socializing, running errands, eating meals, relaxing, or—if you're like some people—catching up on work and so on. You see, you *do* have time to exercise; you just aren't making it a priority.

How can you shift your priorities? First, you've got to make a commitment to yourself and to your health. Realize that if you don't do so, your well-being will continue to be compromised, and—to be perfectly grim—the time you have available to do anything will be up a lot sooner than you think. Your health is your most precious asset; it's time to start treating it as such.

One of the most tried-and-true ways to ensure you make time for exercise is to mark your workouts on your calendar and make them

The**GoalDigger**Tip

Tune out.
If you're going to make time to exercise, something's got to give in your schedule. I'm going to guess that one of the things filling up several hours in your day is one of America's favorite pastimes: television. According to ACNielsen, the average American watches more than 4 hours of TV each day. That's 28 hours a week! If you do this consistently for 65 years of your life, nearly 11 of those years will have been spent in front of the tube. If you absolutely cannot—will not—give up *American Idol* or *Lost* or *CSI* or *Oprah*, I would beseech you to at least get your exercise *while* you watch. This certainly isn't the ideal—I believe a lot of people work less intensely and are less tuned in to their bodies when distracted by television—but it's better than nothing.

a nonnegotiable part of each and every week—appointments that you simply cannot and will not cancel, no matter what comes up. You wouldn't just cavalierly "skip" a meeting with your boss; why would you do it with your most precious asset? I know it sounds like work, but the other important part of this equation is to set your sights on engaging in activities you enjoy. Clearly, we only make time for the things we like to do—so make exercise an enjoyable priority, and I'm certain you'll find you not only have the time to devote to getting in shape, but might actually cancel *other* things in order to work out. You'll simply be feeling so good and having such a great time that your priorities will automatically shift.

Section Three: You're Hurt and Aching (For Excuses to Not Exercise)

If you're suffering from an illness or injury—or simply a body that's no longer as fit as it once was—of *course* it's going to be tough for you to exercise the way you'd like, let alone participate in life in any dynamic way. Few things will stop a person from getting needed activity as quickly as a physical ailment. But at most, such impediments should merely be setbacks—not something that keeps you from being active ever again. After

goaldigger*inspiration*

Sluggish Thirtysomething Loses Weight, Becomes Personal Trainer

One day 38-year-old Emily Renninger of Woodland Hills, California, woke up to discover that the image she had of herself as a "fit girl" had completely disappeared from her reality. "Most of my activity was in the form of walking, yoga, and feeble on-and-off attempts at maintaining a workout regimen at the gym," Renninger recalls. "Then, in my mid-30s, I realized I had actually put on 30 pounds and almost stopped regular activity altogether. I knew something had to change and fast!"

But, eager as Renninger was to get back in shape, she took things at a sensible pace. She began by enrolling in Weight Watchers and shed 20 pounds before rejoining a gym, where she signed on to work with a personal trainer once a week. "I knew if I was going to accomplish my goal of reclaiming 'fit girl' once and for all, I needed help," Renninger explains. "I started slowly, and as I gained confidence and knowledge, I began adding a day at a time to my routine. Before I knew it, I was seeing results and had gained a new understanding of the entire process." So much so that Renninger actually became a certified trainer herself!

While she admits that she suffered from lagging motivation and energy at

all, if you don't address your aches and pains or whatever it is that's plaguing your health, these problems will only persist and, ultimately, get worse.

If you're truly determined to reclaim your fitness and kick it up a notch (and I assume you are if you're reading this book!), then that's the best reason you could have to see a doctor and get the treatment you need. In most cases, I believe, any medical professional will advise you to ease back into an exercise program and gradually rebuild your fitness foundation. From there, it's only a matter of time before you start feeling better and all those health problems you were experiencing become less of an issue, if they even continue at all. As I'm sure you know, exercise is not the enemy in these situations; movement and activity will be your ticket to better health and get you

---

first, Renninger dug deep and found reasons to commit for good. "I started looking at this as my last shot," she says. "After all, I wasn't getting any younger and didn't want to find myself 40 and fat." By listening to her body, she found even more motivation. "If I fell off the wagon, I paid attention to how I felt, physically and mentally," Renninger recalls. "If I had a few bad days of eating poorly, I realized I didn't feel good. If I missed a few days at the gym, I noticed how sluggish I was. Before long, exercise was such a normal part of my routine that I started scheduling things around my workouts rather than putting exercise off for other events."

About a year and a half later, Renninger was completely transformed—mentally and physically. "I used to live to eat; now I eat to live," she says. "I used to try something once and give up if it was too hard—now I know just how far I can really push myself and how good if feels to try." Ultimately, Renninger lost over 30 pounds and well over 10 percent body fat—but more important than that, she says: "I gained a new sense of confidence and power that I never knew I had." She now recommends putting in the effort, not only to her clients, but to everyone. "You'll never know how much fight and strength you have within unless you challenge yourself," she says. "When you do, you'll find a sense of pride and accomplishment that is unequaled."

back to your previous activity level or an even higher one—no matter what your starting point.

If you think you're too old and weary, think again: Only through activity will you rediscover your youth and vitality. There's a saying I love: "We do not stop playing because we grow old; we grow old because we stop playing." In other words, perhaps your inactivity is precisely the reason you got hurt or are suffering aches and pains and feeling old and creaky in the first place.

Bottom line: Consult with your doctor and start working on correcting your physical problems. You may be referred to a physical therapist, a personal trainer who specializes in specific types of diseases and ailments, or even someone like a chiropractor. There are so many specialists who can help you get your body back on track, and then the sky's the limit as far as how much exercise you'll be capable of doing. (For more on preventing illness and injury before it strikes and treating it in a worst-case scenario, turn to Chapter 6.)

Section Four: Your Motivation Is as Weak as Your Excuses

There are people in this world who love to exercise, and then there are others who view being active as a necessary evil. You obviously fall into the latter category at the moment, and there are a number of possible reasons why your apathy has escalated.

First, you may have started looking at working out as something you *have*

The**GoalDigger**Tip

Look on the dark side.

Do you feel like exercise is something you have to do, rather than something you want to do? In such situations, I often advise people to think about how they would feel if they suddenly lost the use of their legs or any other part of the body. Practically every time I work out, I do this. When I imagine what it would be like to be completely paralyzed, I'm instantly grateful for every last thing my body is capable of doing—and that's when I really give the workout my all. Suddenly, I'm not burdened by having to move; an inability to move would really be the burden—wouldn't it?

The**GoalDigger**Tip

Dig deep.

If your motivation to move is waning, maybe your reasons for doing it aren't big or specific enough. As you'll see in the next chapter, goal-setting is an important way to keep yourself going—and you need to be incredibly detailed, realistic, and ambitious about what you want. So start thinking about that now: What do you want to accomplish with exercise? Can you picture the changes you'd like to see in your body (beyond the numbers on the scale)? Are there physical feats you want to be able to perform (like running a 5K or even a marathon)? Do you want to be able to play with your kids more energetically, or have more passion for your work, or live to see your 50th wedding anniversary? Turn to the Goal Digger Log on page 183 and start recording the most compelling reasons you can think of for exercising, and in no time you'll be looking forward to the process of getting there.

to do in order to be healthy, lose weight, or achieve any number of fitness goals. While this is certainly true, it's not exactly the most motivating way of looking at it, is it? When you think of being active as an obligation, you not only put a lot of pressure on yourself to do it but beat yourself up if you don't. So it's time to shift your perspective, perhaps back to where it was months or even years ago. For me, it comes down to realizing that exercise is an opportunity and privilege—something I *get* and *want* to do. (Don't think being able to engage in physical activity is an opportunity and privilege? Imagine being paralyzed from the waist down.)

That brings me to the second possible reason for your exercise ennui: You're thinking of being active as work rather than play. Of course you won't want to do it if it feels like a job! That's why you've got to explore a variety of activities, find something you'll actually look forward to doing, something you can genuinely say you like and appreciate being able to do. When you were a kid, I imagine, every opportunity to be active was a thrill. If that was the case, then try to recapture that childlike excitement. By the same token, I know there are people who had bad exercise experiences as children; maybe you were picked last for a game at recess, or there was too much emphasis

The**GoalDigger**Tip

Find a strong personal trainer.

Looking for a professional to help you reach your fitness goals can be an exercise in frustration—but it doesn't have to be. Just make sure you do your homework, and don't go with the first person recommended to you. Interview each prospective personal trainer before hiring anyone to make sure you like his or her personality and training style—and to get details on educational background and areas of expertise. Your trainer should hold a degree (at least a bachelor's but ideally a master's or even a doctorate) in a health- or fitness-related field such as exercise physiology or physical education *and* at least one certification from an accredited organization. That little word *accredited* is very important because just about anyone these days can do a quickie Internet course and get certified—meaning the person you hire might not be properly educated. I recommend looking for certification from the American Council on Exercise (ACE), the American College of Sports Medicine (ACSM), and/or the National Strength and Conditioning Association (NSCA), all of which have impeccable standards and require their trainers to get continuing education on a regular basis and sign a code of ethics. Visit the organizations' Web sites to find certified trainers in your area at www. acefitness.org, www.acsm.org, and www.nsca-lift.org.

placed on winning at a particular sport rather than simply playing for the fun of it. Again, this goes hand in hand with finding things you like to do and doing them, not because you need to excel at them or win at them or have to do them, but merely because they feel good, invigorate you, and make you feel alive.

On that note, a third possible reason for being opposed to exercise is that a lot of workouts are simply not fun for everyone. Frankly, many of them are boring as hell. But one person's hell may be another's heaven. Yes, there are individuals who *love* running on the treadmill for an hour. Others feel this way about doing crunches or circuit-training in the weight room. If those forms of exercise bore you to tears, you need—again—to seek out things that will give you a mental boost and engage you on every level—not just a physical one.

There are a million different ways you can move your body—from hiking to skiing to taking a yoga class to gardening to dancing. I find it hard to believe that every last one of them puts you to sleep. You simply haven't explored enough—so start doing so today. Then, really mix things up, since sticking with only one form of movement day after day will put you on the fast track to tedium—and your body will get stuck in as much of a rut as your mind. Variety is the spice of life, and that's particularly true of exercise. If you used to enjoy being active but don't anymore, perhaps it's because you became too reliant on one particular workout and need to push yourself in a new direction. Set your sights on discovering a new activity weekly, if not daily. Each time you do that activity, play with the variables—whether it's doing it at a different pace, playing with the order of the exercises, moving to different types of music, or working out in different locations. I think you'll soon find that you're more than motivated, and you look forward to exercise each and every time and miss it when you're not doing it.

Section Five: You're in the Dark about Exercise

As I mentioned back in the introduction to this book, a lot of people simply don't know what they should be doing in order to achieve their fitness goals. While you're not alone in that, allowing a lack of knowledge or skills to stop you from realizing your personal best would be nothing short of tragic.

Let me begin by saying there's a very good chance you know a lot more than you think you do—and it's even possible you're making things more complicated than they really are. My advice would be to take that first step—literally. You don't need to enroll in some crazy cardio fusion class at the local gym to achieve a greater level of fitness; simply putting one foot in front of the other—easing yourself into a walking program and then intensifying it from there—may be the perfect initial ticket. It all depends on your starting point. Whatever that is, the secret to boosting your fitness lies in gradually making things more challenging—not in going for something to such an extreme that you feel overwhelmed and even run the risk of hurting yourself.

Beyond this, you should probably get some guidance. If I may be so bold: Reading this book is an excellent place to start. In the next chapter I'm going to help you zero in on your goals, and in the chapter after that, you'll

The**GoalDigger**Tip

Gear up without breaking the bank.

There's no reason to spend a lot of money in your quest for a better body. A good pair of walking or running shoes should run you only $60 to $80 (look for brands like Asics, Nike, and Saucony). If swimming is more your speed, a suit needn't cost more than $40, while goggles run about $5 to $27 (find some good ones at www.sealmask.com). Something like cycling could be more costly but still reasonably affordable; bikes range in price from $600 to $3,000 (check out Scott bikes at www.scottusa.com), and helmets cost around $50 (look for Rudy Project at www.erudy.com or Bell at www. bellhelmets.com).

Working out at a fitness facility doesn't have to put you in debt either. Find out if there's a YMCA near you, where rates are often quite low— particularly when the entire family joins. (Hey, if it was good enough for the Village People, shouldn't it be for you too?) Some colleges and universities also allow the public to use their gyms for reasonable rates and are worth investigating.

If you're more of a homebody and have the space, there's no reason you can't find affordable equipment. An indoor bike trainer can cost as little as $80 (check out Cycleops at www.cycleops.com) or as much as $1,000 or more (visit Computrainer at www.racermate.com). If you absolutely love—

discover a variety of programs that won't just help you achieve those goals but will also be tailored specifically to your experience *and* energy levels, as well as your available time.

That said, I'm not so egomaniacal to think that this book is the be-all and end-all of your quest for knowledge. In fact, if you feel like you're not sure about what you're doing—on any level—when it comes to exercise, it's *imperative* that you get some professional help. No, I'm not telling you to see a shrink—I'm saying you should enlist the help of a well-qualified and motivating personal trainer. If you don't know what you're doing, you won't just compromise your fitness results but could actually wind up with an injury. Let me put it this way: When you don't know how to get your finances in

and I mean love—elliptical trainers or treadmills, then I recommend purchasing one because you will likely use it. Steer clear of the cheapest models; they're no fun to use and may not even challenge you sufficiently. But you don't have to go for the most expensive machines either. Get a middle-of-the-line machine and you'll be fine. My favorite product line for ellipticals, treadmills, and bike trainers is Precor (www.precor.com)—and they have a good range of prices for just about every budget.

As for strength equipment, you don't necessarily need to pay big bucks for a Bowflex. A set of dumbbells can cost anywhere from $100 to $300 (Powerblocks are terrific: www.powerblock.com), depending on how many you need, and resistance tubing is just $10 apiece (check out www.spriproducts.com). These tools, along with others we'll talk about in Chapter 4, allow you to perform dynamic, functional, multimuscle exercises that can be just as challenging, if not more so, than the isolation moves typically done with machines. Shop around at sporting goods stores (especially secondhand ones), and I'm sure you can outfit a home gym for a pretty reasonable chunk of change. And hey, some great strength gains can be made by using your own body weight: Pushups and situps can be performed anywhere—and they are indeed extremely effective.

order, you go to an accountant. Getting your body in order should be no different. Seek out an expert who can show you the best possible way to achieve your fitness goals, and you'll probably reach them more swiftly and safely. (For more details on what to look for in a personal trainer, see the box on page 14.)

Section Six: You're Environ-Mental

When you decide you want to boost your fitness and really take things to the next level, you may think you need a ton of new equipment and gear or a fancy facility decked out with the most expensive machines money can buy, or that any adverse circumstances—like weather or a hectic travel schedule or a carbuncle on your foot—will throw your training off course. All of these factors only serve to leave you feeling like you've got the will but not the way. Wrong.

Just like people who aren't quite sure what they need to do to reach their fitness goals, you're probably making things a lot more complicated than they need to be. As you'll see in Chapter 3, workouts that deliver significant results don't require much in the way of equipment. In fact, a lot of the most beneficial and challenging strength moves are the ones that use your own body weight as resistance, while some of the most effective aerobic activities are basic routines involving walking, jogging, swimming, and the like. How much expensive equipment do these things require? Next to none. Plus, you can do them inside, outside, almost anywhere—so you can't claim crummy weather or being out of town as outs.

Didn't Score in Any Section?

If you didn't score five points in any of the six sections on the previous pages—well, either you're not being honest with yourself ... or I've completely lost touch with the most common excuses people have for not exer-

TheGoalDiggerTip

Seek support.

Want to know one of the single best excuse-busters on the planet? Other people. Seriously, *immediately* start surrounding yourself with individuals who will support you in your quest to boost your fitness. All you need to do is tell your friends, family, coworkers, training buddies, or other fitness professionals (like a personal trainer, if you decide to go that route) that you want to get in better shape and make exercise a priority in your life. Tell them you've decided you're going to do this, once and for all. Then ask if they'd be willing to call you on your excuses whenever you try to wiggle out of your commitment. Anytime you're about to back out of a workout, call one of these people to discuss why. You might just find that the mere thought of telling someone else your excuse is enough to make you see how invalid it is in the first place ... and you'll get moving without even telling your supporter(s) you were going to bail. Game over, game on.

The**GoalDigger**Tip

Be your own worst critic.

If you want to stop your perceived obstacles dead in their tracks, get out a pen and paper and write down a list of each and every excuse (beyond the ones in this chapter) that you personally have for not exercising. Then, as I've done, start making a list of all the reasons these aren't *really* obstacles, and brainstorm ways you can actually overcome them. Be tough on yourself! In doing so, you'll ultimately come out ahead.

cising ... or you're simply psyched up and ready to go. My hope is that it's the latter.

Either way, now that we've got all those excuses out of the way, it's time to get started—to home in on what you want to achieve, without anything standing in the way of your success. You're unencumbered and ready to go!

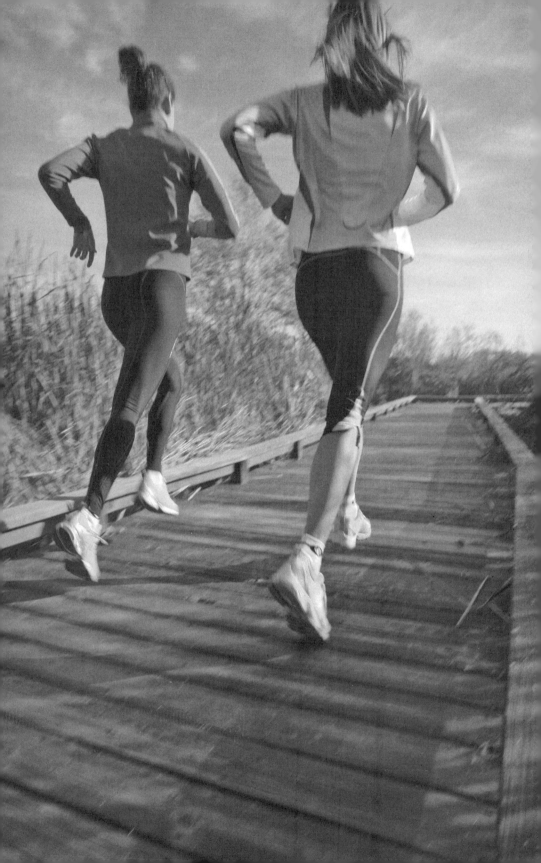

TWO

Digging for Goals: Discover What You Want and Why You Want It

"So what'cha, what'cha, what'cha want?"
—**Beastie Boys**

"Many persons have the wrong idea of what constitutes true happiness. It is not attained through self-gratification but through fidelity to a worthy purpose."
—**Helen Keller**

Okay, so Mike D (Michael Diamond), MCA (Adam Yauch), and Adrock (Adam Horovitz) of the Beastie Boys and Helen Keller are an odd pairing, but these quotes together sum up what it means to have true, mission-driven goals.

Now that you're past all the excuses and obstacles standing in the way of you seriously kicking butt, you may feel like there's a light at the end of the

< 21 >

tunnel, shining brightly on what you want to accomplish—but is there? You know what they say about opinions and a certain part of your anatomy: Everybody's got one. The same is true of fitness goals. Just about everyone you encounter will be able to tell you why they work out (or why they would if they did), whether it's to lose a few pounds, pummel a pal on the racquetball court, blow off steam after a stressful day, or keep a particular ailment in check. The simple fact that you're reading this book means you obviously have a goal, or a few of them, in mind.

But let's be honest: How clearly can you identify what you want? How specific can you get? If things are sort of fuzzy and vague, that could be an even bigger obstacle than the ones addressed in the last chapter. Why? Because you're shooting blind with no target in sight; you don't really know

The**GoalDigger**Tip

Make your goal the action, not the outcome.

Wanting to look better, feel better, perform better, achieve optimum health—these are all worthwhile and highly motivating pursuits and are absolutely going to be the end result when you kick your training into high gear. But these things are also more difficult to track from one day and workout to the next. So I suggest that in addition to these outcome-oriented goals, you pinpoint the steps that you'll take to achieve those things and make those your shorter-term goals. The 14-Day Programs in the next chapter are great for that, because each workout within each plan can be your goal for the day. But what's possible beyond that?

There are plenty of specifics you can shoot for, from a target number of exercises or sets or reps or weight in a particular strength-training workout to a specific duration or intensity for your cardio workouts to longer-term actions like running a marathon. That's how Dana Villamagna, 33, of Appleton, Wisconsin, approached her goal of losing the pregnancy pounds after having each of her three children. Yes, she wanted to lose weight, but her goals were also to train for a marathon after the first baby, a triathlon after the second, and a half-marathon after the third—and she achieved what she set out to do on all counts. Turn to page 28 for her full story.

what's driving you or the deep-seated reasons you'll be putting in the time, day after day. You simply cannot become a goal digger athlete without very specifically pinpointing your mark. You need to develop a crystal-clear picture of what you want. From there, you'll be able to figure out how realistic it is and what kind of program will get you there, as well as setting short-term goals along the way so you can measure your progress effectively.

In this chapter, you're not just going to get to the bottom of what you want to achieve in your fitness program—you're going to prioritize every last goal. You're also going to address why you're setting your sights on these results, what you stand to gain by achieving them, and what else might be motivating you. Only in doing these exercises can you figure out how to get where you're going while staying consistent, focused, and inspired. In Chapter 3, I'm going to provide you with detailed workout programs tailored to what you want to accomplish. Beyond being goal-specific, these plans will have additional variables, which I'll show you how to modify according to your abilities and experience level, your available time, and even your energy levels on any given day.

Better yet, each of these programs requires only an initial 14-day commitment. After that, you can either repeat the plan until you reach your specified target or retake the Goal Digger survey below to determine if—and how—your priorities and goals may have shifted (and they very well may) and modify your program accordingly. But let's not get ahead of ourselves. First we need to figure out what'cha, what'cha, what'cha want! Ready to do some soul-searching? Then let's begin!

THE GOAL DIGGER SURVEY

What are your reasons for exercising—and what do you want your workouts to accomplish? The statements in each section below will help you determine that. As you read though them, think about how strongly each one resonates with you, and rate it on a scale from zero ("not important to me at all") to 10 ("extremely important to me").

SECTION ONE

[10] I want to lose weight.

[10] I want to look less flabby.

10 I want to appear more toned and muscular.

10 I want to reduce the size of my waist, hips, butt, and/or other areas.

10 I want to burn as many calories as possible.

10 I want my clothes to fit better.

10 I want to look good in a swimsuit.

8 I want to look younger (or like I used to look).

10 I want to improve my posture—to appear longer and leaner.

10 I just want to like the reflection I see in the mirror.

98 **TOTAL FOR THIS SECTION**

SECTION TWO

10 I want to feel more energetic.

10 I want to blow off steam.

10 I want to reduce my stress levels.

10 I want to feel a sense of accomplishment.

10 I want greater confidence.

10 I want to have more passion for life.

10 I want to feel more awake and alert.

10 I want to have more balance in my life.

10 I want to keep things in a healthier perspective.

10 I want to be happier.

100 **TOTAL FOR THIS SECTION**

SECTION THREE

10 I want to participate or improve in an athletic event or sport.

10 I want to channel my competitive fire.

10 I want to move faster.

10 I want to boost my endurance.

[10] I want to increase the duration of my workouts.

[10] I want to get stronger and/or more muscular.

[10] I want a serious adrenaline rush.

[10] I want to challenge myself.

[10] I want to push my limits.

[10] I want to win!

[100] **TOTAL FOR THIS SECTION**

SECTION FOUR

[10] I want to live a long life.

[10] I want to minimize or prevent aches, pains, and/or injuries.

[10] I want to ward off illness and disease.

[10] I want to minimize fatigue.

[10] I want to be sharper and more focused.

[10] I want to feel younger, more vital.

[10] I want to decrease my body fat percentage.

[10] I want to build my lean muscle mass.

[10] I want to lower my body mass index (BMI).

[10] I want to be healthier in every way.

[100] **TOTAL FOR THIS SECTION**

SO HOW DID YOU DO? We'll get to that in a moment. First, let's consider the survey you just completed and point out something that may or may not be obvious: When it comes to exercise, the payoffs are vast—and regardless of what you say you want to accomplish, you're going to wind up getting a lot more than you bargained for in the process. If you lose weight, you boost your health, energy, and ability to perform at your peak. If you exercise for better health, chances are you're going to wear a smaller clothing size and boost your energy and ability to perform. If all of these things are important to you, then there's a good chance you scored high marks in every category—and not only is that okay, it's great! It simply means you're aware of all you stand to gain from taking your fitness to the next level, and now you just need to prioritize and hone those goals until you can feel them in your bones. These are the things that are going to be motivating you and that you need to stay inspired, to push yourself as far as you can possibly go. Now let's talk about each goal in greater detail.

YOUR RESULTS

The section in which you scored highest will be your primary goal and will determine the first 14-Day Program you perform, as set forth in the next chapter. After completing said program, you may choose to repeat it for another 14 days, or you may return to this chapter and reassess your goals. If you scored high—or the same number—in more than one section, it's up to you to determine which goal resonates most deeply with you and with what you want, first and foremost, from the program you're about to take on. Read through the sections in which you scored highest to further solidify what you want, then turn to Chapter 3, where I'll show you how to get there. Now let's break it down by category.

Section One

If you scored highest in this section, your primary goal is to LOOK BETTER.

No doubt about it: We live in an appearance-obsessed world, and getting a buffed-up, slimmed-down, superhot physique is certainly a huge driving force behind millions of resolutions to exercise, time and again. Setting your sights on getting ripped or svelte can be incredibly motivating. After all, the harder you work, the more results you'll see, from a jiggle-free butt to better posture to more comfortable—even smaller—clothes to an allover healthy glow. Meanwhile, looking good and feeling good go hand in hand; when you like what you see in the mirror, you're more confident, you have more energy, you want to exercise ... and when you're more confident, have more energy, and want to exercise, you'll inevitably look fabulous, dahling.

That's all the good stuff. Now for the reality check: When you exercise to lose weight or improve your appearance, results may vary—and they'll take some time to show up. I certainly don't need to tell you that genetics plays a role (in spite of the magazines that swear you can get Jessica Simpson's butt in 8 weeks flat) or that a six-pack and sculpted thighs aren't going to appear overnight. Beyond all this, the scale rarely reflects what's happening to your

The**GoalDigger**Tip

Get wise about weight loss.

Perhaps you've noticed America's obsession with thinness, which has been fanatically furthered by the media. Yet in spite of all the ways we fixate upon and revere the supremely skinny, we are collectively fatter than ever. Maybe if we stopped idealizing a size-zero physique and instead promoted healthy and realistic weight goals, obesity (and crash dieting and eating disorders) would be almost obsolete.

So what's a realistic and healthy weight for you? The body mass index (BMI) is one way to determine that number (see the chart on page 33)—although it doesn't take certain factors into account, like age, sex, and body composition. Other factors worth considering include a healthy waist circumference and body fat percentage (both also noted in the chart). My suggestion: Simply shoot for the weight at which you feel healthiest, happiest, and most energetic. Even more important: Make sure you don't take it off too quickly. Two pounds a week is considered the absolute maximum amount you should lose if you're doing things safely and sensibly and to ensure it stays off for good.

body, especially in the short term, so if you're pinning your hopes on a number, you may be in for some disappointment. Perhaps these are some of the reasons you've let your fitness regimen fade to black—and all the more reason you need to further hone your goals.

Yes, the Look Better 14-Day Program in the next chapter is designed to boost your metabolism, burn maximum calories, and deliver relatively fast results (particularly when combined with the eat-right strategies in Chapter 7), but the aesthetic transformation will happen gradually. So, beyond improving your appearance or achieving some magic number on the scale, you're going to need to put pen to paper and fill in some more solid details—sort of like a motivational road map that will help you get to your destination. Why do you want to achieve a better body, and what do you want beneath and beyond that? That's what the Goal Digger Log on page 183 will help you determine. Go there now, then turn to Chapter 3 to get rolling with the 14-Day Look Better Program.

(continued on page 30)

Former High School Runner Competes in Marathons and Triathlons to Lose Pregnancy Pounds— And Gains a Whole Lot More

Dana Villamagna, 33, of Appleton, Wisconsin, is a prime example of someone who has set her sights on specific action- *and* outcome-oriented goals—and between that and being realistic about her wants and abilities, she has successfully resurrected the fire of the athlete within. The action: competing in athletic events. The outcomes: weight loss, better health, setting an example for her kids, raising money for a worthy cause, and consistently increasing her fitness.

Villamagna, who once ran cross-country in high school, is now a writer and mother of three children (ages 8, 4, and 1) who found that each of her pregnancies took a toll on her body and her ability to be active. "I gained 50 to 75 pounds with each baby and couldn't work out—except for yoga—due to extreme morning sickness," Villamagna explains. "So after giving birth, I would set a goal for myself [first child: marathon, second: triathlon, third: half-marathon] and whip myself back into shape. The adage 'nine months up, nine months down' held true for me."

But Villamagna's training didn't just help her to lose the baby weight. "During one perilous time when I had an ectopic tubal pregnancy, I nearly lost my life and had to have multiple blood transfusions," she says. "The doctor said having just trained for a marathon and being in top condition saved my life when my blood supply was so low."

It's maintaining that level of fitness—along with setting short- *and* long-term goals—that further fuels Villamagna's motivation. "Now that baby number three is nearly 1 year old, I've decided to train for another half-marathon, with an additional goal of decreasing my time by 30 minutes from the last race," Villamagna says. "I've also set long-term goals for myself of completing a half-Ironman by age 37 and an Ironman triathlon by age 40."

That's not to say there haven't been obstacles. "Finding time to get in good, solid workouts is tough," says Villamagna. "As a mom and a writer, I always have things come up that knock me off my planned training times." She relies on help from her husband (a recent medical school graduate who's now a resident), uses the YMCA's childcare facilities while she works out, and hires a babysitter when necessary. Keeping track of her goals is crucial to her success as well. "I wrote my short-term and long-term goals down on paper—on the same paper as my professional and our family goals, giving them importance for the whole family—and I look at them daily to remind myself what I'm trying to achieve and why," Villamagna says.

She also stresses that being realistic about her abilities and goals is of utmost importance. "When I was in high school, I ran to the extreme (100 miles in a week one summer!), but now I accept my own personal limitations," she notes. "I'm a finisher, not a competitor; being real about my age and my limitations as a busy mom has actually helped me reach my goals and keep working at an appropriate fitness level. My best friend is a triathlete. She wins races in her age group and qualifies for all kinds of elite events. When I do my Ironman event, I'll be finishing in the dark when most people have already gone home! But I will finish. That's the reality, and that's what's important to me."

Regardless of where she finishes in the races she trains for, the victories Villamagna enjoys are many. "Physically, I feel great," she says. "I can also fit into my favorite pair of tattered and torn size six jeans that I've had since college. My writing is taking a new twist, and my life feels more integrated." Meanwhile, she and her 8-year-old daughter raised more than $11,000 for the Leukemia and Lymphoma Society when she ran her last half-marathon.

Bottom line: By setting the goal of competing in athletic events, Villamagna has achieved more than most everyday athletes might ever imagine. "A life in which all of my goals and daily activities are connected in some way with my family, my accomplishments, and my spiritual path is critical to my success," Villamagna concludes. "Until I realized that my health and fitness were part of that integrity, I would always fall short. Now that I see the benefits—spiritually, physically, mentally, professionally, and within my marriage and family—of keeping these goals in mind, I will remain committed."

Section Two

If you scored highest in this section, your primary goal is to FEEL BETTER.

Like a lot of people, you've probably become run-down and weary, if not downright bitter, as a result of a fast-paced, hectic lifestyle. So what's your bastion of hope, the one thing that will help you recapture your energy and approach every day with a positive outlook and less stress? Exercise! Lucky for you, achieving these things could be as little as one workout away—and that may be reason enough for you to stick with it time and again.

However, it's crucial that you train your body in ways that will maximize your energy levels and mood. If you're not feeling 100 percent and then try to push your body to the limit, it's very likely it will stage a mutiny, and you'll wind up far more exhausted and drained than you'd expected. Even if you are feeling great but overtrain, things could take a turn for the worse (we'll talk more about this in Chapter 6). That's why you'll be assessing your physical abilities before embarking on any of the programs in the next chapter, as well as gauging your energy levels prior to every workout you do. If you don't have the power to give the program your all, I'll show you how to modify it so you'll still reap the desired rewards. Of course, diet is also an important part of the energy equation. Turn to Chapter 7 for tips on how many calories you should be consuming and what types of foods will best fuel your exercise and keep you on an even keel from one day to the next.

The**GoalDigger**Tip

Address your energy crisis.

Research shows that exercise can help combat chronic fatigue syndrome—but if you're tired all the time and find that activity still leaves you exhausted, see your doctor to rule out any underlying medical conditions such as thyroid disease or anemia. Also, make sure you're eating enough (calories are energy, and if you're crash dieting you're going to crash; see Chapter 7 for more on the importance of consuming enough calories), that you're getting an adequate amount of sleep (7 to 9 hours a night, per the National Sleep Foundation), and that you're doing whatever you can to minimize stress in your life. Taking certain vitamins, like an iron supplement or a B-complex that includes B_6, may also help.

I encourage you to keep track of your mood and energy levels as you put the workouts in Chapter 3 into practice, whether you continue with the Feel Better Program or switch over to another goal. I particularly recommend that you write down how you're feeling before and after each training session (there's room to do so in your daily workout log, which you can find on page 194), as well as on the days you don't exercise. I think you'll quickly find that you not only achieve everything you hope for on the days you train, but that your energy levels slump if you skip a few days.

And finally, as with every goal, I suggest you elaborate upon all the reasons you want to take your training to the next level, above and beyond how it will make you feel. What else do you want to accomplish: What's driving you to take the next step, and how are you going to get there? The more detailed you can get and the more reasons you can find for working out, the more motivated you'll be. Turn to the Goal Digger Feel Better Log on page 186 and spend some time thinking about every last ambition you have, then flip to the 14-Day Feel Better Program in Chapter 3 and get the boost you're after.

Section Three

If you scored highest in this section, your primary goal is to PERFORM BETTER.

Whether you're looking to get an edge over your competition in a particular athletic endeavor or simply achieve your own personal best, regular and challenging training sessions are crucial. And while keeping your eyes on the prize will help you stay focused on getting your game where you want it to be, there's more to it than that.

In order to see improvement in your physical abilities, you're going to need to monitor things closely. Starting your program with a fitness test (as you'll do in Chapter 3, prior to beginning your 14-Day Perform Better Program) will help you gauge where your strengths and weaknesses lie—and will help you track your progress. Meanwhile, you'll want to make sure you're doing the right balance of activities and not pushing yourself so hard that you wind up hurting yourself. The Perform Better Program takes all of this into account (and Chapter 6 further addresses various ways to make sure you're exercising safely). Getting enough calories, in the right balance of nutrients, is also of paramount importance; you'll find more details about fueling your body for maximum performance in Chapter 7.

Now, while competition—even if it's simply with yourself—can provide an extreme amount of motivation, I firmly believe that you can go even deeper and find additional reasons for embarking upon the program outlined in the next chapter. As with all of the fitness goals addressed here, I'd like you to take some time to think about why you've set this goal for yourself and what else is at stake for you. The Goal Digger Perform Better log on page 188 will push you to figure out every last one of your motivators, so when you get started in Chapter 3, victory will be yours!

Section Four

If you scored highest in this section, your primary goal is BETTER HEALTH.

First, allow me to commend you for making this your mission, for it is perhaps the best possible reason to exercise. The evidence simply cannot be denied: When you're sedentary, you risk all kinds of ailments and injuries.

The**GoalDigger**Tip

Get your vitals, stat.

Taking your fitness to the next level doesn't just require proper diet and exercise; regular medical checkups and screening tests are also an important part of the equation. Here's a rundown of some of the most important health exams and how often to get them.

BLOOD PRESSURE TEST: **At least every 2 years**

BONE MINERAL DENSITY TEST: **At age 65; repeat as directed by a physician**

CHOLESTEROL TEST: **At age 20, then every 5 years**

DIABETES/BLOOD SUGAR TEST: **At age 45, then every 3 years**

THYROID TEST: **At age 35, then every 5 years**

For additional information on when to get various checkups, preventive screening tests, and immunizations, visit www.4woman.gov/ screeningcharts (which provides links to informational charts for both women and men).

What's Your BMI?

Body mass index, or BMI, is your weight in kilograms divided by your height in meters squared. The table below has already done the math and metric conversions. To use the table, find your height in the left-hand column, then move across the row to find your weight. The number at the top of the column is the BMI for that height and weight.

BMI (KG/M2)	19	20	21	22	23	24	25	26	27	28	29	30	35	40
HEIGHT (IN)	WEIGHT (LBS)													
58	91	96	100	105	110	115	119	124	129	134	138	143	167	191
59	94	99	104	109	114	119	124	128	133	138	143	148	173	198
60	97	102	107	112	118	123	128	133	138	143	148	153	179	204
61	100	106	111	116	122	127	132	137	143	148	153	158	185	211
62	104	109	115	120	126	131	136	142	147	153	158	164	191	218
63	107	113	118	124	130	135	141	146	152	158	163	169	197	225
64	110	116	122	128	134	140	145	151	157	163	169	174	204	232
65	114	120	126	132	138	144	150	156	162	168	174	180	210	240
66	118	124	130	136	142	148	155	161	167	173	179	186	216	247
67	121	127	134	140	146	153	159	166	172	178	185	191	223	255
68	125	131	138	144	151	158	164	171	177	184	190	197	230	262
69	128	135	142	149	155	162	169	176	182	189	196	203	236	270
70	132	139	146	153	160	167	174	181	188	195	202	207	243	278
71	136	143	150	157	165	172	179	186	193	200	208	215	250	286
72	140	147	154	162	169	177	184	191	199	206	213	221	258	294
73	144	151	159	166	174	182	189	197	204	212	219	227	265	302
74	148	155	163	171	179	186	194	202	210	218	225	233	272	311
75	152	160	168	176	184	192	200	208	216	224	232	240	279	319
76	156	164	172	180	189	197	205	213	221	230	238	246	287	328

When you're active, your chances of living a longer life, while minimizing illnesses and physical impediments, go up considerably. Research consistently shows that regular exercise can help prevent heart disease, obesity, high blood pressure, type 2 diabetes, osteoporosis, and mental health problems such as depression. The key is to exercise frequently and intensely enough—while also doing so in a way that's sensible and beneficial to your

Risk of Associated Disease, according to BMI and Waist Size

BMI		WAIST LESS THAN OR EQUAL TO 40" (MEN) OR 35" (WOMEN)	WAIST GREATER THAN 40" (MEN) OR 35" (WOMEN)
18.5 or less	Underweight	Not applicable	Not applicable
18.5–24.9	Normal	Not applicable	Not applicable
25–29.9	Overweight	Increased	High
30–34.9	Obese	High	Very high
35–39.9	Obese	Very high	Very high
40 or greater	Extremely obese	Extremely high	Extremely high

SOURCE: The National Institutes of Health

body. (Diet plays an important role as well, which we'll address in Chapter 7.) The 14-Day Better Health Program in the next chapter is designed to help you on all of those counts.

I do have to admit, though, I've met more than a few people who have said that exercising to be healthy just isn't motivating enough for them. A lot of these people are on the younger side and feel they've got their whole lives ahead of them, that they are immune to illness and injury; frankly, they've got an immortality complex. Well, let me tell *you* something, young whipper-snappers … Seriously, my guess is that if your primary goal has to do with being healthy and injury free, you may have already experienced something of a wake-up call, whether it was a difficult diagnosis or some physical damage. I hope this isn't the case, but if it is, then I need to encourage you to seek the advice of a physician before commencing the program in the next chapter (as everyone should before beginning any new workout).

In the event that you are perfectly healthy and simply want to stay that way, I'd still encourage you to take a look at the reasons you've set this goal—and to explore what else is driving you to exercise. Why? As the people who aren't motivated enough by this goal will tell you, "better health" isn't exactly something you notice when you're already functioning pretty well (and even when you're not); you're preserving something that people often take for granted until it's no longer there. (In the words of Joni Mitchell: "Don't it always seem to go that you don't know what you've got till it's gone.") So setting your sights on things you can track in no uncertain terms will keep you all the more inspired. On the other hand, if you're starting out with high blood pressure, depression, or any number of ailments and your doctor's given you the okay to go forward with the 14-Day Feel Better Program, you'll definitely be able to track your progress—in hard numbers and in the way you feel.

Regardless of why you've made health your top priority, I urge you to take a look at the Goal Digger Feel Better Log on page 186 and map out exactly what your concerns are and how you'd like to see them improve (with specific numbers if you've got them), as well as any other goals you have beyond physical fitness. Then you'll be ready to begin your program in Chapter 3. I'm excited to see just how great you feel after only 14 days.

Now that you've figured out which program best matches your psychology and taken some time to fill out the applicable Goal Digger log(s), it's time to address your physiology and your daily schedule. What are you capable of achieving? What's realistic within the context of your life? Turn to the next chapter to find out.

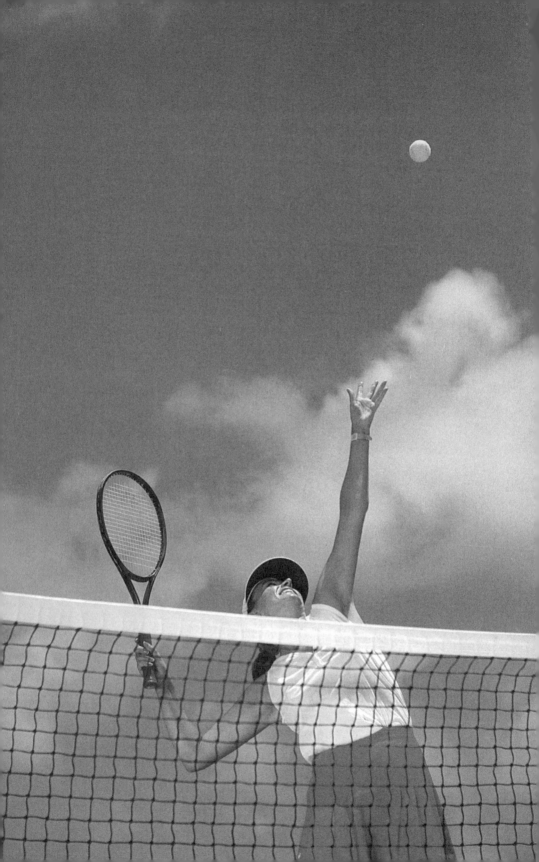

THREE

Go for It! The 14-Day Programs

"The human body is made up of some 400 muscles, evolved through centuries of physical activity. Unless these are used, they will deteriorate."
—Eugene Lyman Fisk

"It is exercise alone that supports the spirits and keeps the mind in vigor."
—Cicero

So you've set your goals and determined exactly what's driving you toward them. You're motivated, your eyes are fixed on your target, and now you're ready for the exercise prescription that's going to get you there. That prescription will be coming at you momentarily—and I think you'll find that these programs not only deliver the results you're after, but do so in a way

< 37 >

that keeps you revved and ready for more. Why? Rather than prescribing a 6- or 14-week program, which can feel daunting, you'll only have to commit to an entirely doable—and enjoyable—14-day "miniplan." (And you can even get several days off!) Research shows that people have little trouble adhering to exercise for 14 days; it's the period after that when significant attrition occurs. These programs will show you just how manageable it can be to take your workouts to new heights, and my bet is you'll want to continue with a second program and a third and so on. Before you know it, you'll find 6 or 10 weeks isn't so daunting after all—and you want to keep going for good!

We just need to take into account a few more factors, above and beyond your goals. That's because these programs aren't based only on the results of the Goal Digger surveys you completed in the previous chapter; they will be further customized according to your current fitness level, available time, and energy levels on any given day. Once we've got all this information, you'll be able to get rolling. Let the final countdown—and your final preexercise exams—begin!

TEST #1: ARE YOU EXPERIENCED?

First off, we're going to get a read on your current fitness level. Perhaps you used to compete on a superhuman level; maybe you've been exercising consistently for the past few months or more; there's even a chance you've been challenging yourself on occasion. Then again, perhaps you haven't been doing much of anything that could qualify as bona fide, heart-pumping, muscle-building activity in ages. While your athletic background and recent workout patterns might be applicable here, in order to prescribe the best possible program for you, we need to assess how fit you are right now—today. Therefore, you're going to have to do some actual exercise—a self-test of sorts. Hey, it will be fun. After all, don't you want to know how fit you are and then keep track of how much progress you make? Of course you do!

So get out your walking or running shoes (that's all the equipment you'll need) and take the following strength and cardiovascular fitness tests. These will help you determine whether you should do the beginner, intermediate, or advanced workouts designed for your goal. After you complete your 14-Day Program (and every subsequent one), I recommend retaking the tests to see how your score has improved—and whether it's time to move to the next level. My bet is you'll be cranking things up in no time flat. But why stop at the advanced level? If and when you're really rocking and need an even greater challenge, simply turn to the next chapter, where I'll show you still more ways to maximize your results—without putting in any extra time. For now, though, let's move on to the fitness tests.

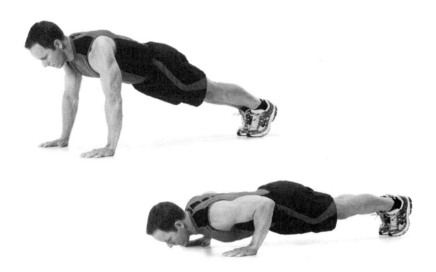

Upper-Body Strength Test

Do as many pushups as you can, continuously and with perfect form (no time limit), and record the number on the scorecard on page 42.

HOW TO PERFORM A PUSHUP

1. Support your body with the balls of your feet and your hands, positioning your hands about 3 inches more than shoulder-width apart on either side, palms flat on the floor. Straighten your arms without locking your elbows. Your butt should be slightly above the line of your body so your back doesn't sag.

2. Lower your torso until your chest is almost to the floor. Push yourself up to the starting position and repeat.

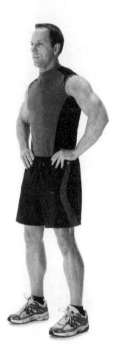
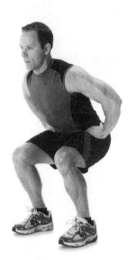

Lower-Body Strength Test

Do as many squats as you can in 1 minute, continuously and with perfect form, and record the number on the scorecard on page 42.

HOW TO PERFORM A SQUAT

1. Stand with your hands on your hips and your feet shoulder-width apart. Keep your shoulder blades back and your toes pointed straight ahead.

2. Initiating your descent at the hips, not the knees, lower yourself as though sitting into a chair (making sure to go no lower than the point where your thighs are parallel to the floor). Keep your lower back in its natural alignment, and avoid moving your knees forward past your toes. Return to the starting position by standing as you push down through your heels, and repeat.

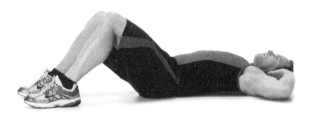

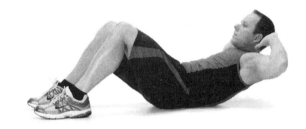

Abdominal Strength Test

Do as many crunches as you can in 1 minute, continuously and with perfect form, and record the number on the scorecard on page 42.

HOW TO PERFORM A CRUNCH

1. Lie on your back with your knees bent and your feet flat on the floor, about hip-width apart. Place your fingertips lightly behind your ears to gently support your head.

2. Use your abs to lift your head and shoulder blades 4 to 6 inches off the floor. Keep your lower back pressed firmly against the floor and your elbows pointing straight out (not forward). Hold as you exhale, then slowly lower back to the starting position, and repeat.

Cardiovascular Strength Test*

Walk, jog, or run as fast as you comfortably can—either on flat terrain or on a treadmill set at zero incline—and when you hit 1.5 miles, record your time on the scorecard below. Be sure to warm up and cool down with 5 to 10 minutes of easy walking (but do not count that distance as part of the 1.5 miles or include those minutes in your total time)—and don't eat anything 2 hours prior to taking this test. Also, don't push yourself *too* hard; you want to do well, but you don't want to make yourself sick just for the sake of your score!

Fitness Level Scorecard

UPPER-BODY STRENGTH TEST

Number of pushups: _____

LOWER-BODY STRENGTH TEST

Number of squats: _____

ABDOMINAL STRENGTH TEST

Number of crunches: _____

CARDIOVASCULAR STRENGTH TEST

Time: _____

* Based on the Cooper Institute's Aerobic Fitness Test

Your Results

To determine the program you should begin with, find the fitness test in which you scored lowest and use that as your starting point. So, if you're a 25-year-old woman and were able to do 50 crunches and 12 squats but only 4 pushups and 13 minutes on your cardio test, you should start with the intermediate rather than advanced goal-specific program and build from there.

WOMEN

FITNESS LEVEL	AGE: UNDER 20	AGE: 21–35	AGE: 36–45	AGE: 46 AND OVER
BEGINNER	0–5 pushups 0–9 squats 0–25 crunches 13:50+ cardio	0–3 pushups 0–6 squats 0–20 crunches 14:15+ cardio	0–2 pushups 0–4 squats 0–15 crunches 14:45+ cardio	0–1 pushup 0–3 squats 0–10 crunches 15:15+ cardio
INTERMEDIATE	6–15 pushups 10–16 squats 26–50 crunches 10:46–13:49 cardio	4–10 pushups 7–10 squats 21–40 crunches 11:31–14:14 cardio	3–5 pushups 5–8 squats 16–30 crunches 12:16–14:44 cardio	2–4 pushups 4–6 squats 11–20 crunches 12:46–15:14 cardio
ADVANCED	16+ pushups 17+ squats 51+ crunches 10:45 or less cardio	11+ pushups 11+ squats 41+ crunches 11:30 or less cardio	6+ pushups 9+ squats 31+ crunches 12:15 or less cardio	5+ pushups 7+ squats 21+ crunches 12:45 or less cardio

MEN

FITNESS LEVEL	AGE: UNDER 20	AGE: 21–35	AGE: 36–45	AGE: 46 AND OVER
BEGINNER	0–25 pushups 0–16 squats 0–35 crunches 13:20+ cardio	0–20 pushups 0–12 squats 0–30 crunches 13:45+ cardio	0–15 pushups 0–8 squats 0–25 crunches 14:15+ cardio	0–10 pushups 0–6 squats 0–15 crunches 14:45+ cardio
INTERMEDIATE	26–40 pushups 17–24 squats 36–60 crunches 10:16–13:19 cardio	21–30 pushups 13–18 squats 31–50 crunches 11:01–13:44 cardio	16–25 pushups 9–12 squats 26–40 crunches 11:46–14:14 cardio	11–20 pushups 7–10 squats 16–25 crunches 12:16–14:44 cardio
ADVANCED	41+ pushups 25+ squats 61+ crunches 10:15 or less cardio	31+ pushups 19+ squats 51+ crunches 11:00 or less cardio	26+ pushups 13+ squats 41+ crunches 11:45 or less cardio	21+ pushups 11+ squats 26+ crunches 12:15 or less cardio

Now you know your fitness level, you're almost ready to go. But before you proceed, you'll need to assess how you're feeling—and how much time you have available—each day. Then do the corresponding workout within your goal-oriented program.

TEST #2: ARE YOU AMPED?

First, note whether each of the following statements is true or false for you.

1. I'm well rested. True/False

2. I'm not experiencing any aches or pains. True/False

3. I feel moderately, if not supremely, energetic. True/False

4. I'm ready to give my workout at least 80 percent. True/False

5. I want to sweat! True/False

If three or more of the above questions were true for you, you're geared up and ready to do the Challenge Program.

If three or more of the above questions were false for you, begin with the Energize Program. If you feel great after the first 10 minutes of that program, switch over to the Challenge one.

TEST #3: ARE YOU AVAILABLE?

This one's pretty simple, as tests go. You'll have two final options within each program: a Full-Fledged [FF] plan and a Time-Saver [TS] version. Simply look at the FF workout prescribed for any given day, and if you can't possibly make the time for it, opt for the shorter [TS] version. See? I told you it would be easy.

GETTING STARTED

Now that we've considered your goals, energy levels, and available time, you're just about ready to commence your completely customized program. But first, let's go over the components essential to absolutely every workout you'll do.

THE WARMUP

I know, I know: You don't have time to warm up. You're putting in enough effort as it is, and skipping this crucial part of your program just means you're psyched up and ready to rock your workout, right? Wrong. Regardless

The**GoalDigger**Tip

Plan ahead.

Staying well hydrated and well fueled prior to exercise will ensure you perform at your peak during your workouts—but timing is everything on both counts. Two hours before you exercise, try to drink 16 to 24 ounces of water. At least 1 hour prior to working out, have a light snack that's a good balance of protein, fat, and carbohydrates, such as a turkey or peanut butter sandwich and a glass of milk. (This will stabilize your insulin levels and provide you with longer-lasting energy.) Have another 16 ounces of water 10 to 15 minutes before you exercise, and continue to hydrate yourself as needed throughout your workout session. (For more on nutrition, see Chapter 7.)

of the kind of exercise you'll be doing, you *must* start out with at least a few minutes of light aerobic activity—preferably 5 to 10 minutes. This serves to boost your body temperature, effectively priming your muscles and making them better equipped to handle the ass-kicking workout you're about to embark upon. In fact, you'll kick even more ass (rather than getting your ass kicked) if you warm up first, and some experts say you'll even reduce your risk of injury. So prior to every workout in your 14-Day Program, warm up—whether you take a brisk walk on the treadmill before hitting the weights or simply begin your aerobic exercise with 5 to 10 minutes of the same activity at an easy pace.

THE COOLDOWN

Yet another neglected but essential component of the workout, cool down at the end of every exercise session with 5 minutes of low-intensity aerobic activity and stretching to safely bring your heart rate down to its preexercise level. Experts note that stopping too suddenly may cause blood to pool in your arms and legs, preventing it from returning to the heart fast enough and causing lightheadedness and dizziness, while stretching your muscles after both cardio and strength training improves flexibility, helps prepare your body for the next workout, and speeds the body's recovery process, according to the American Council on Exercise. Aim to end each workout with 5 to 10 minutes of light aerobic activity, followed by stretches for all the muscles you just worked. For stretches for specific muscle groups, see pages 86 to 95.

THE CARDIO WORKOUTS

No matter which goal-specific program you do, you'll perform 2 or 3 days of strength training (details in the programs themselves) and 4 or 5 days of cardiovascular exercise each week. The cardio workouts will vary in intensity and duration, which you can track by using a heart rate monitor and/or the more subjective rate of perceived exertion (RPE) scale. See "How to Monitor Your Intensity" on page 48 for more about both methods. Now for the workouts ...

Training Zone 1—steady state: When you do any of these aerobic workouts, you should be exercising at 50 to 60 percent of your maximum heart rate (MHR), and your RPE should be between 10 and 12. This zone builds aerobic fitness, strengthens immunity, and uses your body fat as the primary source of fuel. When instructed to do a steady-state cardio activity in this zone, simply exercise at a nice, steady pace for the duration. (For exam-

The**GoalDigger**Tip

Listen to your body.

After warming up for your workout—but prior to launching into your full session—take a few moments to assess how your body is feeling. This is the listening phase of your exercise, and it's crucial. If your body is feeling warm, energized, and ready to go, you might consider doing a more challenging workout than you'd originally planned (for example, perhaps you were going to do the Energize Program, but now realize you're more up for the Challenge than you'd anticipated). However, if your body is feeling sluggish—even sore—and your breathing isn't coming easily, you may need to go for a less challenging workout, or even skip it altogether. Paying attention to the cues from your body will help you stay motivated and injury free. Just make sure you're listening to the messages coming from your *body* and not those that may be lingering in your mind about things you'd rather be doing (like curling up with a book and a box of chocolates).

ple, hike or bike on fairly even terrain, approaching a somewhat challenging pace but not overtaxing yourself.) You should never feel out of breath when performing a Zone 1 workout.

Training Zone 2—long intervals and tempo: If instructed to exercise in this zone, you'll be "comfortably challenged" at an RPE of 13 to 15, or a heart rate at 60 to 70 percent of your maximum. You'll push yourself, but not to an extreme, boosting your endurance and ability to work at a more challenging pace. The "long intervals" in this zone will entail pushing yourself to RPE 15, or 70 percent of your MHR for 3 to 8 minutes, then recovering completely before pushing yourself again. For instance, you might run two laps and then walk until your heart rate comes back down, then repeat. When your program calls for a "tempo" workout in this zone, push yourself to a slightly less challenging pace (RPE 13, or 60 percent of your MHR) for the duration. (Don't worry—it will be a much shorter period of time!) For Zone 2 workouts, your breathing should feel fairly labored.

The**GoalDigger**Tip

Fuel down.

Yes, exercise is supposed to energize you—but if you feel a little spent after your workouts, it's probably because your blood sugar levels have dropped. This is due to the fact that when you exercise, your muscles use carbohydrate fuel called glycogen. What can you do? Replace that lost fuel with 30 to 50 grams of carbohydrates (try two bananas, a bagel, or an energy bar), along with about 16 ounces of water, as soon after your workout as possible. This will ensure that your exercise leaves you feeling as pumped up as it should. (For more on nutrition, see Chapter 7.)

THE 14-DAY LOOK BETTER PROGRAM

Perhaps you want to lose some weight, or sculpt a more balanced, toned, and beautiful physique, or get a beach-worthy midriff. This program can help you achieve all of that and more. The aerobic cardio workouts will help you lose bodyfat, while the strength moves will shape, tone, and tighten your body. For this program to really work, you need to focus on both elements: the cardio and the strength. Don't give short-shrift to either one. Follow this program and you'll be thrilled with how terrific you look!

(continued on page 50)

How to Monitor Your Intensity

HEART RATE

According to the American College of Sports Medicine, your aerobic workouts should ideally be conducted at between 60 and 90 percent of your maximum heart rate (MHR). If you go beyond 90 percent, you're going to be hating life—and exercise. When you stay in the 60 to 90 percent range, you burn a significant amount of calories and boost your cardiovascular fitness without the risk of overexertion or injury.

How do you determine your ideal heart rate range? You first need to know your MHR. That number is influenced by a variety of factors, including your age, genetics, fitness level, and overall health—but for our purposes, I suggest you estimate it by subtracting your age from 220. (So, if you're 35, your estimated MHR is 185.) Write that number here: _____

Now that you know your MHR, you'll be able to aim for your ideal training zones as prescribed in the cardio workouts. When exercising in Training Zone 1, for example, you should be at 50 to 60 percent of your MHR. So if your maximum is 185 beats per minute, your heart rate should be between 92 and 111 beats per minute during a Training Zone 1 workout ($185 \times 0.5 = 92.5$ and $185 \times 0.6 = 111$).

THE RATE OF PERCEIVED EXERTION

Your target heart rate is an objective measurement of how hard your body is working, but, as previously noted, you can also monitor your exercise intensity in a more subjective way. In 1982, Gunnar Borg, PhD, developed a scale for monitoring intensity based on how hard you feel you're working. The rate of perceived exertion, or RPE, scale provides a quantitative rating of exercise effort. To determine your RPE, just do a brief mental scan of your body while working out—then use the following scale to give your "exercise effort" a number.

RPE SCALE

6
7—very, very light exertion: Something akin to getting up from the couch—hey, it's a start!
8
9—very light exertion: You're hardly working.
10
11—fairly light exertion: You're just beginning to sweat.
12
13—somewhat hard exertion: Breathing is becoming more difficult.
14
15—hard exertion: You begin to feel your muscles exerting themselves.
16
17—very hard exertion: Speaking is a challenge.
18
19—very, very hard exertion: Speaking is impossible.
20

For every cardio workout you do, you can use the target heart rate, the RPE scale, or both.

The Strength Moves

The strength moves in this program are designed to sculpt your entire body and firm up trouble zones. You'll be doing them "circuit-style," which cranks up the calorie burn a notch to help you get lean as you boost your strength and endurance. To perform one circuit, you'll do the number of reps recommended, then move quickly to the next exercise. Completing one set of each move in rapid succession constitutes one "circuit." On the days when you're instructed to do more than one circuit, rest for 2 minutes before cycling through all the strength moves again.

The**Strength**Moves

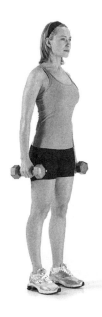
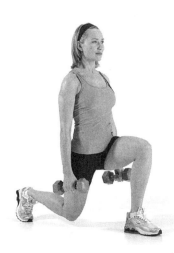

Lunge

Strengthens and sculpts all lower-body muscles, including the quadriceps, hamstrings, buttocks, upper hips, and inner thighs

1. Stand holding two dumbbells at your sides, your feet shoulder-width apart, and your toes pointing straight ahead.

2. Take a large stride forward, far enough so that your front thigh ends up parallel to the floor with your knee over (not past) your toes. Push back up to the starting position by bringing your front leg to your back leg. This motion strengthens your entire leg (and your butt) while increasing the range of motion in your hips—a dynamite exercise. Do 12 repetitions with the first leg and then 12 with the other leg; that's one set. Then move right to the next exercise. (As with all the moves here, use weights that "significantly challenge" you in the last few repetitions of each set, and increase the weight as you grow stronger.)

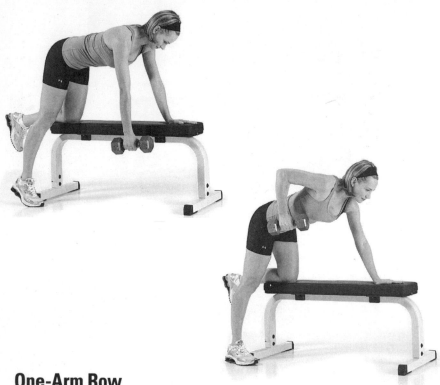

One-Arm Row

Strengthens upper back, shoulders, and arms

1. Holding a dumbbell in your right hand, place your left hand and knee on a workout bench or the seat of a chair. Keep your back flat, and let the dumbbell hang down at your side so that it's just in front of your shoulder.

2. Focus on using your upper-back muscles as you pull the dumbbell up and back toward your hip, keeping your arm close to your body. Do not lift the dumbbell higher than hip level. Pause at the top of the move, then slowly lower the dumbbell to the starting position. Do 12 reps with your right arm and 12 with your left. Then move right to the next exercise.

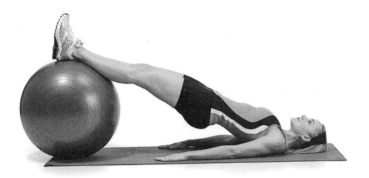

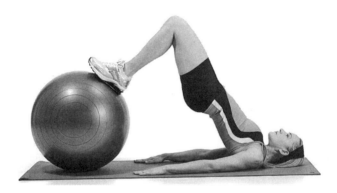

Stability Ball Leg Curl

Strengthens hamstrings, buttocks, abdominals, and lower back

1. Lie on your back on a carpeted floor or an exercise mat with your legs extended and your heels up on a stability ball (balancing on these large inflatable balls strengthens many muscles at once). Keep your arms straight out at your sides, with your palms down. Press down through your heels on the ball to lift your pelvis, butt, and most of your back off the floor. Your body should form a bridge from your shoulder blades to your feet, and you should feel the exertion in the muscles along the backs of your thighs and in your midsection.

2. Keeping your body lifted, squeeze your gluteal muscles and press your feet flat into the ball as you bend your knees and roll the ball in toward you. Pause, then roll the ball back out to the bridge position. Roll the ball in and out 12 times. Then move right to the next exercise.

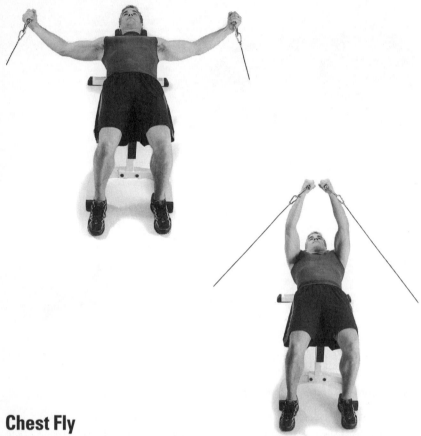

Chest Fly

Strengthens chest, shoulders, and back

1. Sit in a chest-fly machine with your feet a comfortable distance apart and flat on the floor. Grab the handles with a false grip (thumb on the same side as your fingers). Your elbows should be at shoulder height, resting on the pads.

2. Keeping your back and shoulder blades against the backrest, use your chest muscles to squeeze the pads together in front of your chest. Pause before returning to the starting position. Do 12 repetitions. Then move right to the next exercise.

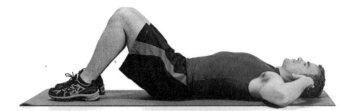

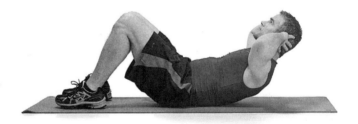

Crunch

Strengthens the abdominals

1. Lie on your back with your knees bent and your feet flat on the floor, about hip-width apart. Place your fingertips lightly behind your ears to gently support your head.

2. Use your abs to lift your head and shoulder blades 4 to 6 inches off the floor. Keep your lower back pressed firmly against the floor and your elbows pointing straight out (not forward). Hold a tight crunch for 10 to 15 seconds as you exhale, then slowly lower back to the starting position. Rest for 15 seconds. Now you've completed one circuit. If instructed, repeat the entire circuit again beginning with the Lunge on page 51.

BEGINNER ENERGIZE PROGRAM

MONDAY FF: Perform cardio workout (e.g., steady walk or hike) for 45 minutes in Training Zone 1. **TS:** Perform cardio workout (e.g., swim, bike, run, vigorous walk or hike) for 20 minutes.

TUESDAY FF: Perform two full circuits of the 5 strength moves as instructed, going quickly from one exercise to the next. Rest for 2 minutes between circuits. **TS:** Perform only 1 circuit.

WEDNESDAY: OFF

THURSDAY FF: 45 minutes cardio, Zone 1, and 2 strength circuits; **TS:** 20 minutes cardio and 1 circuit

FRIDAY FF: 45 minutes cardio, Zone 2; **TS:** 20 minutes cardio

SATURDAY: OFF

SUNDAY FF: 60 minutes cardio, Zone 1; **TS:** 30 minutes cardio

MONDAY: OFF

TUESDAY FF: 45 minutes cardio, Zone 2, and 2 strength circuits; **TS:** 20 minutes cardio and 1 circuit

WEDNESDAY FF: 60 minutes cardio, Zone 1; **TS:** 20 minutes cardio

THURSDAY: OFF

FRIDAY FF: 90 minutes cardio, Zone 1; **TS:** 30 minutes cardio

SATURDAY FF: 3 strength circuits; **TS:** 2 circuits

SUNDAY: OFF

BEGINNER CHALLENGE PROGRAM

MONDAY FF: 45 minutes cardio (e.g., run or bike ride) in Training Zone 2; **TS:** 30 minutes cardio (e.g., swim or vigorous hike/jog)

TUESDAY FF: 60 minutes cardio, Zone 1, and 2 strength circuits; **TS:** 30 minutes cardio and 1 circuit

WEDNESDAY: OFF

THURSDAY FF: 45 minutes cardio, Zone 2; **TS:** 20 minutes cardio

FRIDAY FF: 75 minutes cardio, Zone 1, and 1 strength circuit; **TS:** 30 minutes cardio and 1 circuit of 3 strength moves of choice (shorter circuit today only)

SATURDAY: OFF

SUNDAY FF: 60 minutes cardio, Zone 2, and 1 strength circuit; **TS:** 20 minutes cardio and 1 circuit

MONDAY: OFF

TUESDAY FF: 45 minutes cardio, Zone 1, and 2 strength circuits; **TS:** 20 minutes cardio and 1 circuit

WEDNESDAY FF: 45 minutes cardio, Zone 2; **TS:** 20 minutes cardio

THURSDAY: OFF

FRIDAY FF: 90 minutes cardio, Zone 1; **TS:** 30 minutes cardio

SATURDAY FF: 2 strength circuits; **TS:** 1 circuit

SUNDAY: OFF

INTERMEDIATE ENERGIZE PROGRAM

MONDAY FF: Perform cardio workout (e.g., steady walk or hike) for 45 minutes) in Training Zone 1. **TS:** Perform cardio workout (e.g., moderately vigorous walk, jog, or swim) for 20 minutes.

TUESDAY FF: Perform two full circuits of the 5 strength moves as instructed, going quickly from one exercise to the next. Rest for 2 minutes between circuits. **TS:** Perform only 1 circuit.

WEDNESDAY: OFF

THURSDAY FF: 45 minutes cardio, Zone 1, and 2 strength circuits; **TS:** 20 minutes cardio and 1 circuit

FRIDAY FF: 30 minutes cardio, Zone 2; **TS:** 15 minutes cardio

SATURDAY: OFF

SUNDAY FF: 60 minutes cardio, Zone 1; **TS:** 30 minutes cardio

MONDAY: OFF

TUESDAY FF: 45 minutes cardio, Zone 2, and 2 strength circuits; **TS:** 20 minutes cardio and 1 circuit

WEDNESDAY: 60 minutes cardio, Zone 1; **TS:** 20 minutes cardio

THURSDAY: OFF

FRIDAY FF: 90 minutes cardio, Zone 1; **TS:** 30 minutes cardio

SATURDAY FF: 3 strength circuits; **TS:** 2 circuits

SUNDAY: OFF

INTERMEDIATE CHALLENGE PROGRAM

MONDAY FF: 60 minutes cardio (e.g., run or bike ride) in Training Zone 2; **TS:** 30 minutes cardio (e.g., swim or vigorous hike/jog)

TUESDAY FF: 75 minutes cardio, Zone 1, and 2 strength circuits (8–10 reps); **TS:** 45 minutes cardio and 1 circuit

WEDNESDAY: OFF

THURSDAY FF: 60 minutes cardio, Zone 2; **TS:** 30 minutes cardio

FRIDAY FF: 90 minutes cardio, Zone 1, and 1 strength circuit; **TS:** 30 minutes cardio and 1 circuit of 3 strength moves of choice (shorter circuit today only)

SATURDAY: OFF

SUNDAY FF: 75 minutes cardio, Zone 2, and 1 strength circuit; **TS:** 30 minutes cardio and 1 circuit

MONDAY: OFF

TUESDAY FF: 60 minutes cardio, Zone 1, and 2 strength circuits; **TS:** 30 minutes cardio and 1 strength circuit

WEDNESDAY FF: 60 minutes cardio, Zone 2; **TS:** 30 minutes cardio

THURSDAY: OFF

FRIDAY FF: 2 hours cardio, Zone 1; **TS:** 30 minutes cardio

SATURDAY FF: 2 strength circuits; **TS:** 1 circuit

SUNDAY: OFF

ADVANCED ENERGIZE PROGRAM

MONDAY FF: Perform cardio workout (e.g., steady walk or hike) for 60 minutes in Training Zone 1. **TS:** Perform cardio workout (e.g., moderately vigorous walk, jog, or swim) for 30 minutes.

TUESDAY FF: Perform two full circuits of the 5 strength moves as instructed, going quickly from one exercise to the next. Rest for 2 minutes between circuits. **TS:** Perform only 1 circuit.

WEDNESDAY: OFF

THURSDAY FF: 60 minutes cardio, Zone 1, and 2 strength circuits; **TS:** 30 minutes cardio and 1 circuit

FRIDAY FF: 45 minutes cardio, Zone 2; **TS:** 30 minutes cardio

SATURDAY: OFF

SUNDAY FF: 90 minutes cardio, Zone 1; **TS:** 45 minutes cardio

MONDAY: OFF

TUESDAY FF: 60 minutes cardio, Zone 2, and 2 strength circuits; **TS:** 30 minutes cardio and 2 circuits

WEDNESDAY FF: 75 minutes cardio, Zone 1; **TS:** 30 minutes cardio

THURSDAY: OFF

FRIDAY FF: 2 hours cardio, Zone 1; **TS:** 45 minutes cardio

SATURDAY FF: 3 strength circuits; **TS:** 2 circuits

SUNDAY: OFF

ADVANCED CHALLENGE PROGRAM

MONDAY FF: Perform cardio workout (e.g., run or bike ride) for 90 minutes in Training Zone 2. **TS:** Perform cardio workout (e.g., swim or vigorous hike/jog) for 45 minutes.

TUESDAY FF: 90 minutes cardio, Zone 1, and 3 strength circuits; **TS:** 45 minutes cardio and 1 circuit

WEDNESDAY: OFF

THURSDAY FF: 75 minutes cardio, Zone 2; **TS:** 30 minutes cardio

FRIDAY FF: 2 hours cardio, Zone 1, and 1 strength circuit; **TS:** 45 minutes cardio and 1 circuit of 3 strength moves of choice (shorter circuit today only)

SATURDAY: OFF

SUNDAY FF: 90 minutes cardio, Zone 2, and 1 strength circuit; **TS:** 45 minutes cardio and 1 circuit

MONDAY: OFF

TUESDAY FF: 75 minutes cardio, Zone 1, and 2 strength circuits; **TS:** 30 minutes cardio and 1 circuit

WEDNESDAY FF: 75 minutes cardio, Zone 2; **TS:** 30 minutes cardio

THURSDAY: OFF

FRIDAY FF: 2½ hours cardio, Zone 1; **TS:** 60 minutes cardio

SATURDAY FF: 2 strength circuits; **TS:** 1 circuit

SUNDAY: OFF

THE 14-DAY FEEL BETTER PROGRAM

This program emphasizes mindful exercise, with a focus on getting outdoors for cardio activities that have fluid, continuous movements—to refresh, renew, and reinvigorate you, inside and out. Focus on breathing during your exercise. Stay loose and balanced. Allow any stress you're carrying to "melt away" with every breath during the cardio workouts. In this program, let your body be your guide: for example, if you're midway through a workout and you feel like you're dragging yourself just to finish, then by all means, cut the workout short. This is a "feel better" program; there is no need to push yourself unnecessarily to get through workouts. After all, you're not training for an Ironman here! Finally, choose activities that you really enjoy. For example, if you simply loathe the treadmill, please stay off of it during this program! A better option would be to take a 10-minute drive to a beautiful park or trail for your run (it's well worth the time). I guarantee that taking the extra time to ensure your exercise makes you "feel better" will pay enormous dividends over time.

The Strength Moves

The strength component of this program will focus on using your own body weight—and gravity—to build a toned, balanced, and more resilient physique. Activities such as yoga are terrific adjuncts to your aerobic/cardio workouts. I advise you to join a yoga class or purchase an instructional CD or tape for home use. However, I believe group classes, under the watchful eye of a talented instructor, are preferable because they offer more variety and guidance. Having a scheduled group workout each week also boosts motivation and compliance.

Here are three basic yoga moves I'd like you to focus on (please see the photos that follow and make sure you execute each move with a present-minded focus and flawless technique):

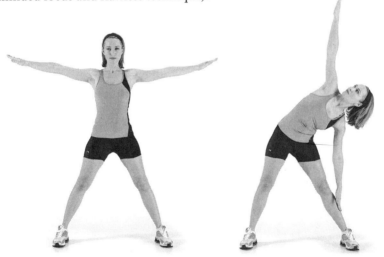

1. **Triangle Pose:** This relatively easy pose strengthens the legs and improves the health of your spine. Spread your feet beyond shoulder-width apart and raise your arms out straight and parallel to the floor. Be sure to keep your knees straight as this allows you to focus on stretching the proper muscles during the pose. While exhaling, perform a slight bend to the left while your left hand slides down toward your left foot—then repeat to the right.

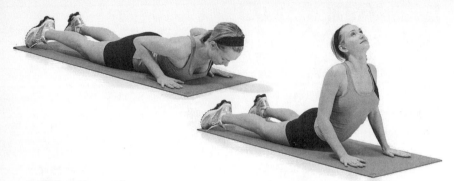

2. **Cobra Pose:** This move opens up the chest as it increases flexibility in the spine. Lie flat on your belly. Then, while exhaling, use your hands (facing forward) to slowly raise your upper body while keeping your hips and legs firmly planted on the floor. As your arms straighten, look upward and back gently and really breathe deeply into the stretch. Your lower back and buttock muscles should be relaxed. You should feel this stretch in the abdominals, upper legs, lower back, and hip flexors.

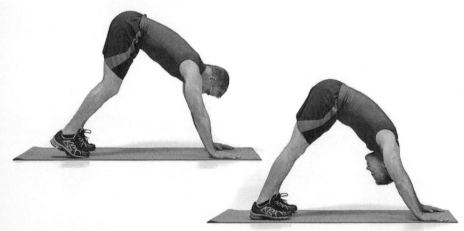

3. **Downward-Facing Dog:** This pose engages virtually all of your muscles, rejuvenating and refreshing you from head to toe. Start with your hands on the ground with your fingers facing forward and your feet at such a distance behind your hands that your body forms a natural "arc." Raise your buttocks into the air and keep your legs straight and your heels pressed firmly into the ground. You should feel the stretch in your upper back and throughout your legs. Make sure to keep your legs straight during this pose and breathe deeply.

BEGINNER ENERGIZE PROGRAM

MONDAY FF: Perform cardio workout (e.g., steady swim or hike outdoors) for 30 minutes in Training Zone 1. **TS:** Perform cardio workout (e.g., moderately vigorous bike ride or swim) for 20 minutes.

TUESDAY FF: Do a 45-minute yoga/Pilates class or home program.
TS: Do 20 minutes of yoga/Pilates

WEDNESDAY: OFF

THURSDAY FF: 30 minutes cardio, Zone 1, and 45 minutes yoga/Pilates;
TS: 20 minutes cardio and 20 minutes yoga/Pilates

FRIDAY FF: 30 minutes cardio, Zone 2; **TS:** 20 minutes

SATURDAY: OFF

SUNDAY FF: 45 minutes cardio, Zone 1; **TS:** 30 minutes cardio

MONDAY: OFF

TUESDAY FF: 30 minutes cardio, Zone 2, and 30 minutes yoga/Pilates;
TS: 30 minutes cardio and 15 minutes yoga/Pilates

WEDNESDAY FF: 45 minutes cardio, Zone 1; **TS:** 30 minutes cardio

THURSDAY: OFF

FRIDAY FF: 60 minutes cardio, Zone 1; **TS:** 30 minutes cardio

SATURDAY FF: 45 minutes yoga/Pilates; **TS:** 20 minutes yoga/Pilates

SUNDAY: OFF

BEGINNER CHALLENGE PROGRAM

MONDAY FF: 45 minutes cardio (e.g., run or bike ride) in Training Zone 2;
TS: 30 minutes cardio (e.g., swim or vigorous hike/jog)

TUESDAY FF: 60 minutes cardio, Zone 1, and 30 minutes yoga/Pilates;
TS: 30 minutes cardio and 15 minutes yoga/Pilates

WEDNESDAY: OFF

THURSDAY FF: 45 minutes cardio, Zone 2; **TS:** 30 minutes cardio, Zone 2

FRIDAY FF: 75 minutes cardio, Zone 1, and 30 minutes yoga/Pilates; **TS:** 30 minutes cardio and 15 minutes yoga/Pilates

SATURDAY: OFF

SUNDAY FF: 60 minutes cardio, Zone 2, and 45 minutes yoga/Pilates; **TS:** 30 minutes cardio and 15 minutes yoga/Pilates

MONDAY: OFF

TUESDAY FF: 45 minutes cardio, Zone 1, and 30 minutes yoga/Pilates; **TS:** 30 minutes cardio and 15 minutes yoga/Pilates

WEDNESDAY FF: 45 minutes cardio, Zone 2; **TS:** 20 minutes cardio

THURSDAY: OFF

FRIDAY FF: 90 minutes, cardio, Zone 1; **TS:** 30 minutes cardio

SATURDAY FF: 45 minutes yoga/Pilates; **TS:** 15 minutes yoga/Pilates

SUNDAY: OFF

INTERMEDIATE ENERGIZE PROGRAM

MONDAY FF: Perform cardio workout (e.g., steady swim or hike outdoors) for 45 minutes in Training Zone 1. **TS:** Perform cardio workout (e.g., moderately vigorous bike ride or swim) for 30 minutes.

TUESDAY FF: Do a 60-minute yoga/Pilates class or home program. **TS:** Do 20 minutes of yoga/Pilates class.

WEDNESDAY: OFF

THURSDAY FF: 45 minutes, cardio, Zone 1, and 45 minutes yoga/Pilates; **TS:** 30 minutes cardio and 15 minutes yoga/Pilates

FRIDAY FF: 45 minutes cardio, Zone 2; **TS:** 30 minutes cardio

SATURDAY: OFF

SUNDAY FF: 60 minutes cardio, Zone 1; **TS:** 30 minutes cardio

MONDAY: OFF

TUESDAY FF: 45 minutes cardio, Zone 2, and 60 minutes yoga/Pilates; **TS:** 30 minutes cardio and 15 minutes yoga/Pilates

WEDNESDAY FF: 60 minutes cardio, Zone 1; **TS:** 30 minutes cardio

THURSDAY: OFF

FRIDAY FF: 75 minutes cardio, Zone 1; **TS:** 30 minutes cardio

SATURDAY FF: 60 minutes yoga/Pilates; **TS:** 30 minutes yoga/Pilates

SUNDAY: OFF

INTERMEDIATE CHALLENGE PROGRAM

MONDAY FF: 60 minutes cardio (e.g. run or bike ride) in Training Zone 2; **TS:** 30 minutes cardio (e.g. swim or vigorous hike/jog)

TUESDAY FF: 75 minutes cardio, Zone 1, and 45 minutes yoga/Pilates; **TS:** 30 minutes cardio and 15 minutes yoga/Pilates

WEDNESDAY: OFF

THURSDAY FF: 60 minutes cardio, Zone 2; **TS:** 30 minutes cardio, Zone 2

FRIDAY FF: 90 minutes cardio, Zone 1 and 45 minutes yoga/Pilates; **TS:** 30 minutes cardio and 15 minutes yoga/Pilates

SATURDAY: OFF

SUNDAY FF: 75 minutes cardio, Zone 2, and 45 minutes yoga/Pilates; **TS:** 30 minutes cardio and 20 minutes yoga/Pilates

MONDAY: OFF

TUESDAY FF: 60 minutes cardio, Zone 1, and 30 minutes yoga/Pilates; **TS:** 30 minutes cardio and 15 minutes yoga/Pilates

WEDNESDAY FF: 60 minutes cardio, Zone 2; **TS:** 30 minutes cardio

THURSDAY: OFF

FRIDAY FF: 2 hours cardio, Zone 1; **TS:** 45 minutes cardio

SATURDAY FF: 60 minutes yoga/Pilates; **TS:** 30 minutes yoga/Pilates

SUNDAY: OFF

ADVANCED ENERGIZE PROGRAM

MONDAY FF: Perform cardio workout (e.g., steady swim or hike outdoors) for 60 minutes in Training Zone 1. **TS:** Perform cardio workout (e.g., moderately vigorous bike ride or swim) for 30 minutes.

TUESDAY FF: Do a 60-minute yoga/Pilates class or home program. **TS:** Do 30 minutes of yoga/Pilates.

WEDNESDAY: OFF

THURSDAY FF: 60 minutes cardio, Zone 1, and 60 minutes yoga/Pilates; **TS:** 30 minutes cardio and 20 minutes yoga/Pilates

FRIDAY FF: 60 minutes cardio, Zone 2; **TS:** 30 minutes cardio

SATURDAY: OFF

SUNDAY FF: 75 minutes cardio, Zone 1; **TS:** 45 minutes cardio

MONDAY: OFF

TUESDAY FF: 60 minutes cardio, Zone 2, and 60 minutes yoga/Pilates; **TS:** 30 minutes cardio and 20 minutes yoga/Pilates

WEDNESDAY FF: 75 minutes cardio, Zone 1; **TS:** 30 minutes cardio

THURSDAY: OFF

FRIDAY FF: 90 minutes cardio, Zone 1; **TS:** 45 minutes cardio

SATURDAY FF: 60 minutes yoga/Pilates; **TS:** 30 minutes yoga/Pilates

SUNDAY: OFF

ADVANCED CHALLENGE PROGRAM

MONDAY FF: 75 minutes cardio (e.g., run or bike ride) in Training Zone 2; **TS:** 60 minutes cardio (e.g., swim or vigorous hike/jog)

TUESDAY FF: 90 minutes cardio, Zone 1, and 60 minutes yoga/Pilates; **TS:** 30 minutes cardio and 30 minutes yoga/Pilates

WEDNESDAY: OFF

THURSDAY FF: 75 minutes cardio, Zone 2; **TS:** 45 minutes cardio

FRIDAY FF: 2 hours cardio, Zone 1, and 60 minutes yoga/Pilates;
TS: 45 minutes cardio and 15 minutes yoga/Pilates

SATURDAY: OFF

SUNDAY FF: 75 minutes cardio, Zone 2, and 60 minutes yoga/Pilates;
TS: 45 minutes cardio and 20 minutes yoga/Pilates

MONDAY: OFF

TUESDAY FF: 60 minutes cardio, Zone 1, and 30 minutes yoga/Pilates;
TS: 30 minutes cardio and 15 minutes yoga/Pilates

WEDNESDAY FF: 60 minutes cardio, Zone 2; **TS:** 30 minutes cardio

THURSDAY: OFF

FRIDAY FF: 2½ hours cardio, Zone 1; **TS:** 45 minutes cardio

SATURDAY FF: 60 minutes yoga/Pilates; **TS:** 30 minutes yoga/Pilates

SUNDAY: OFF

THE 14-DAY PERFORM BETTER PROGRAM

If you are training for any kind of athletic event (5-K walk or run, 10-K run, marathon, bike century, criterium, triathlon … Raid Gauloises!), this is the program for you. You'll be working on challenging your muscles with comprehensive, total-body strength workouts as well as boosting your aerobic fitness (and improving your neuromuscular pathways and biomechanical technique) with higher-intensity workouts. While it's important that you focus almost exclusively on practicing your sport of choice (i.e., running for a marathon), it's a good idea to integrate some cross-training to avoid injury and keep your program fresh.

The Strength Moves

The key to improving your performance in your sport of choice is strengthening the muscles you will be using in said sport—also known as "sport-specific training." For example, if you are training for a marathon, you need to build total-body strength, but with the greatest emphasis on your quadriceps, calves, and hamstrings—the muscles used to power your running stride. Also, in this case you wouldn't want to add muscle size but, rather, build endurance, so you'd stick to higher repetitions (12 to 20). It is beyond the scope of this book to design all the types of sport-specific programs as well as cover individual needs. I recommend that you perform 2 to 3 straight sets of the 5 moves described on pages 51–55 as a foundation—and then work with a certified personal trainer to develop a complete program tailored to you and your sport.

There are so many exercises you can do to improve your performance. Here are just some of the sport-specific moves I would recommend. If you're a . . .

. . . **cyclist:** focus on your quadriceps, lower back, and hamstrings. Three great exercises for these three muscle groups are: leg presses, back extensions, and leg curls.

. . . **runner:** spend extra time on your hamstrings (again with leg curls) and calves (calf raises). Also, strengthen your shins by walking on your heels for a couple minutes after every run.

. . . **swimmer:** your power comes primarily from your back muscles, specifically the latissimus dorsi. Straight armed lat pull-downs are great for swimmers. Stretch Cordz are an excellent "dry-land" training aid, too.

. . . **tennis player:** this is a sport of stops and starts. You must strengthen your hips, knees, and ankles to withstand the lateral pressures. A great tool for this is a Reebok Core Board or a BOSU Balance Trainer.

. . . **basketball player:** work on your calf muscles (with calf raises) and focus on your "core" with abdominal and lower back exercises.

BEGINNER ENERGIZE PROGRAM

MONDAY FF: Perform sport-specific training (e.g., steady run) for 45 minutes in Zone 1. **TS:** Perform sport-specific training (e.g., moderate jog or swim) for 30 minutes.

TUESDAY FF: 45 minutes strength training; **TS:** 20 minutes strength training

WEDNESDAY: OFF

THURSDAY FF: 45 minutes sport-specific training, Zone 2, and 30 minutes strength training; **TS:** 30 minutes sport-specific training and 15 minutes strength training

FRIDAY FF: 45 minutes sport-specific training, Zone 2; **TS:** 30 minutes sport-specific training

SATURDAY: OFF

SUNDAY FF: 60 minutes sport-specific training, Zone 1; **TS:** 30 minutes sport-specific training

MONDAY: OFF

TUESDAY FF: 45 minutes sport-specific training, Zone 2, and 45 minutes strength training; **TS:** 20 minutes sport-specific training and 20 minutes strength training

WEDNESDAY FF: 60 minutes sport-specific training, Zone 1; **TS:** 30 minutes sport-specific training

THURSDAY: OFF

FRIDAY FF: 90 minutes sport-specific training, Zone 1; **TS:** 30 minutes sport-specific training

SATURDAY FF: 45 minutes strength training; **TS:** 20 minutes strength training

SUNDAY: OFF

BEGINNER CHALLENGE PROGRAM

MONDAY FF: 60 minutes sport-specific training (e.g., steady run) in Zone 1; **TS:** 30 minutes sport-specific training (e.g., moderate jog or swim)

TUESDAY FF: 45 minutes strength training; **TS:** 20 minutes strength training

WEDNESDAY: OFF

THURSDAY FF: 60 minutes sport-specific training, Zone 2, and 30 minutes strength training; **TS:** 30 minutes sport-specific training, Zone 2, and 15 minutes strength training

FRIDAY FF: 60 minutes sport-specific training, Zone 2; **TS:** 30 minutes sport-specific training

SATURDAY: OFF

SUNDAY FF: 45 minutes sport-specific training, Zone 1; **TS:** 30 minutes sport-specific training

MONDAY: OFF

TUESDAY: OFF

WEDNESDAY FF: 90 minutes sport-specific training, Zone 1; **TS:** 30 minutes sport-specific training

THURSDAY: OFF

FRIDAY FF: 2 hours sport-specific training, Zone 1; **TS:** 45 minutes sport-specific training

SATURDAY FF: 60 minutes strength training; **TS:** 30 minutes strength training

SUNDAY: OFF

INTERMEDIATE ENERGIZE PROGRAM

MONDAY FF: Perform sport-specific training (e.g., steady run) for 70 minutes in Zone 1. **TS:** Perform sport-specific training (e.g., moderate jog or swim) for 30 minutes.

TUESDAY FF: 60 minutes strength training; **TS:** 30 minutes strength training

WEDNESDAY: OFF

THURSDAY FF: 60 minutes sport-specific training, Zone 2, and 45 minutes strength training; **TS:** 30 minutes sport-specific training and 20 minutes strength training

FRIDAY FF: 60 minutes sport-specific training, Zone 2; **TS:** 30 minutes sport-specific training

SATURDAY: OFF

SUNDAY FF: 75 minutes sport-specific training, Zone 1; **TS:** 30 minutes sport-specific training

MONDAY: OFF

TUESDAY FF: 60 minutes sport-specific training, Zone 2, and 45 minutes strength training; **TS:** 30 minutes sport-specific training and 20 minutes strength training

WEDNESDAY FF: 75 minutes sport-specific training, Zone 1; **TS:** 30 minutes sport-specific training, Zone 1

THURSDAY: OFF

FRIDAY FF: 2 hours sport-specific training: Zone 1; **TS:** 45 minutes sport-specific training

SATURDAY FF: 60 minutes strength-training; **TS:** 30 minutes strength training

SUNDAY: OFF

INTERMEDIATE CHALLENGE PROGRAM

MONDAY FF: 75 minutes sport-specific training (e.g., steady run) in Zone 1; **TS:** 30 minutes sport-specific training (e.g., moderate jog or swim)

TUESDAY FF: 60 minutes strength training; **TS:** 30 minutes strength training

WEDNESDAY: OFF

THURSDAY FF: 75 minutes sport-specific training, Zone 2, and 45 minutes strength training; **TS:** 30 minutes sport-specific training and 20 minutes strength training

FRIDAY FF: 75 minutes sport-specific training, Zone 2; **TS:** 30 minutes sport-specific training

SATURDAY: OFF

SUNDAY FF: 60 minutes sport-specific training, Zone 1; **TS:** 30 minutes sport-specific training

MONDAY: OFF

TUESDAY: OFF

WEDNESDAY FF: 2 hours sport-specific training, Zone 1; **TS:** 45 minutes sport-specific training

THURSDAY: OFF

FRIDAY FF: 2½ hours sport-specific training, Zone 1; **TS:** 45 minutes sport-specific training

SATURDAY FF: 60 minutes strength training; **TS:** 20 minutes strength training

SUNDAY: OFF

ADVANCED ENERGIZE PROGRAM

MONDAY FF: Perform sport-specific training (e.g., steady run) for 75 minutes in Zone 1. **TS:** Perform sport-specific training (e.g., moderate jog or swim) for 30 minutes.

TUESDAY FF: 75 minutes strength training; **TS:** 30 minutes strength training

WEDNESDAY:OFF

THURSDAY FF: 75 minutes sport-specific training, Zone 2, and 45 minutes strength training; **TS:** 30 minutes sport-specific training, Zone 2, and 20 minutes strength training

FRIDAY FF: 75 minutes sport-specific training, Zone 2; **TS:** 30 minutes sport-specific training

SATURDAY: OFF

SUNDAY FF: 90 minutes sport-specific training, Zone 1; **TS:** 30 minutes sport-specific training

MONDAY: OFF

TUESDAY FF: 75 minutes sport-specific training, Zone 2, and 45 minutes strength training; **TS:** 30 minutes sport-specific training and 20 minutes strength training

WEDNESDAY FF: 90 minutes sport-specific training, Zone 1; **TS:** 30 minutes sport-specific training

THURSDAY: OFF

FRIDAY FF: 2½ hours sport-specific training, Zone 1; **TS:** 30 minutes sport-specific training

SATURDAY FF: 60 minutes strength training; **TS:** 20 minutes strength training

SUNDAY: OFF

ADVANCED CHALLENGE PROGRAM

MONDAY FF: 90 minutes sport-specific training (e.g., steady run) in Zone 1; **TS:** 30 minutes sport-specific training (e.g., moderate jog or swim)

TUESDAY FF: 90 minutes strength training; **TS:** 30 minutes strength training

WEDNESDAY: OFF

THURSDAY FF: 90 minutes sport-specific training, Zone 2, and 60 minutes strength training; **TS:** 30 minutes sport-specific training and 20 minutes strength training

FRIDAY FF: 90 minutes sport-specific training, Zone 2; **TS:** 30 minutes sport-specific training

SATURDAY: OFF

SUNDAY FF: 90 minutes sport-specific training, Zone 1; **TS:** 30 minutes sport-specific training

MONDAY: OFF

TUESDAY: OFF

WEDNESDAY FF: 2½ hours sport-specific training, Zone 1; **TS:** 45 minutes sport-specific training

THURSDAY: OFF

FRIDAY FF: 3 hours sport-specific training, Zone 1; **TS:** 60 minutes sport-specific training

SATURDAY FF: 90 minutes strength training; **TS:** 30 minutes strength training

SUNDAY: OFF

THE 14-DAY BETTER HEALTH PROGRAM

This program is designed to help you live longer and better—with more grace and gusto. The strength portion of this program is designed to improve the integrity of your muscles, ligaments, and tendons—in order to prevent injury and reduce any pain you might be feeling. The relaxed nature of cardio workouts will help to boost your immune system. This program only contains Level 1 and Level 2 aerobic workouts, to keep you from overdoing it at all. You should never feel out of breath on the cardio workouts. A well-rounded "better health" program addresses the health of your mind, just as it does the health of your body. Focus on clearing your mind of distracting thoughts during your workouts. Finally, try to do as many of your cardio workouts as possible in beautiful locales; these will bring body benefits and enrich your mind and spirit, too.

The Strength Moves

The keys to any "better health" strength program is to ease into the program, progress slowly—and use excellent form. You don't want your strength work to cause any injuries! Strength moves should be performed smoothly, with a full range of motion and under the watchful eye of a competent trainer. You should focus on deep, relaxed breathing as you strengthen your body. Don't push yourself too hard on this program. And, above all: if something doesn't feel right to you, stop immediately. Your body is a terrific coach, if you just listen to it.

A good strength training program to help you achieve the goal of "better health" is a simple 20-minute "circuit" at your local gym or health club. Choose six machines that you feel comfortable with and that work every major muscle group in the following order (with sample exercises): quadriceps (leg extension), upper back (lat pulldown), hamstrings (leg curl), lower back (low back extensions), calves (calf raise), and abdominals (ab crunch). Do two sets of 15 repetitions on each machine, with 30 seconds of rest

(continued on page 81)

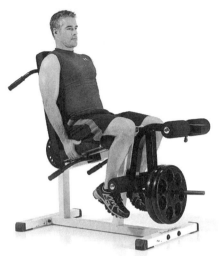

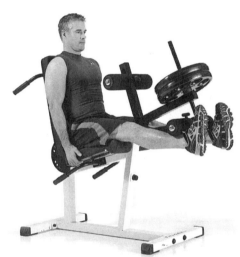

Leg Extension

Quadriceps

1. Adjust the seat so that when you sit down in the machine, your ankles fall behind the ankle pads and your knees line up with the "pivot joint" of the machine. Place your hands on the handles or on the bottom of the seat. Look forward. Keep your back flat against the backrest and your upper body relaxed.

2. As you exhale bring both legs up together in a fluid motion until they are straight out in front of you. In other words, your upper and lower body should form a 90-degree angle. Your toes should point straight up. Pause for a moment and then lower the weight gently back to the starting point.

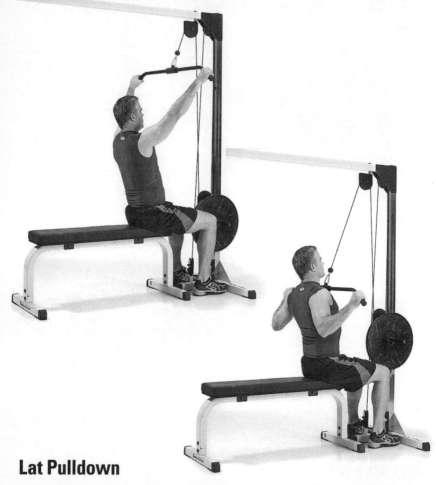

Lat Pulldown

1. Sit directly in front of the lat pulldown machine with your feet flat on the floor, and grab the bar with a comfortable grip about 6 inches wider than shoulder-length on both sides. Keep your arms straight and your torso upright or leaning back slightly. Your back should remain straight, not arched.

2. Pull your shoulder blades together and down, stick out your chest, and pull the bar down toward your chest. Pause with the bar just past your chin just grazing your chest, and then slowly let it rise to the starting position.

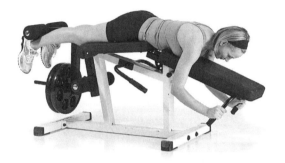

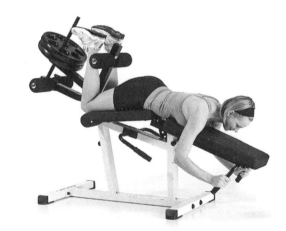

Leg Curl

Hamstrings

1. Lie facedown on the bench of a leg curl machine, with your feet hooked behind the lifting pads and your knees just over the bench's edge. For support, hold on to the bench or the machine's handlebars, if available. Your legs should be fully extended with some flex at the knee and your toes pointing down.

2. Keep your pelvis pressed against the bench as you raise both heels up toward your butt so that your legs bend to a 90-degree angle. Keep your toes pointing out away from your body. Slowly lower your legs back to the starting position. Be sure to exhale as you lift and relax your lower back.

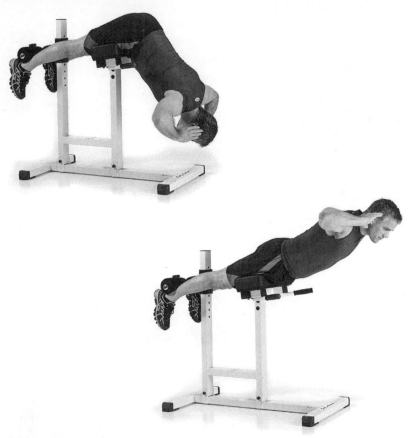

Lower Back Extension

1. Place your hips squarely on the pad and hook your ankles under the foot pad. Slowly lower your body to the starting position and place your hands gently on your ears. In that starting position, your lower and upper body should form a 90-degree angle.

2. Now, engage your lower back muscles and, in a smooth, fluid motion, use those muscles to lift your upper body until it forms a straight line with your lower body. Pause momentarily at the top, then return slowly and carefully to the starting position. Take care not to overextend your back at the top position or overstretch your lower back at the bottom position.

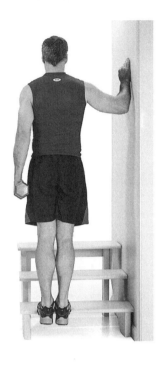

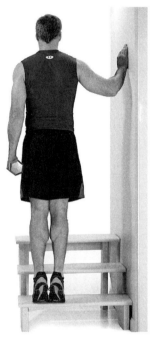

Standing Calf Raise

1. Stand on the bottom step of a staircase, holding a dumbbell in one hand. Hold on to the railing or the wall with your free hand for support. If your home doesn't have a staircase, you can stand on an aerobic step or thick phone book and hold on to the back of a chair at your side. Place the front of both feet on the step so that the balls of your feet are on the step's edge and your heels hang off the back below the level of the step.

2. Keeping your body in a straight line with your toes, lift up onto your toes as high as you can, making sure not to turn your ankles out as you rise. Keep your knees soft (not locked) and avoid leaning forward. Pause in the raised position, and then slowly lower your heels below the level of the step.

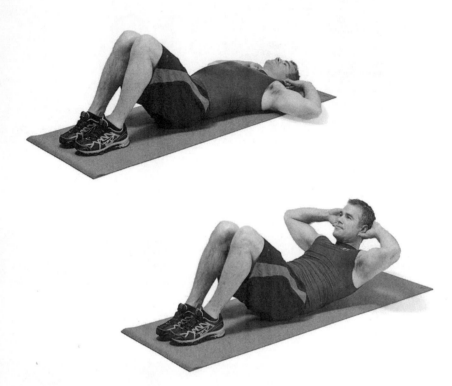

Abdominal Crunch

1. To perform the perfect crunch, lie on your back with your knees bent and your feet flat on the floor about hip-width apart. Place your fingertips lightly behind your head to gently support it.

2. Use your abs—not your arms!—to lift your head and shoulder blades 4 to 6 inches off the floor. Keep your lower back pressed firmly against the floor and your elbows pointing straight out (not forward). Hold a tight crunch for 10 to 15 seconds as you exhale, then slowly lower back to the starting position.

(continued from page 74)

between each set. You should always feel like you're "comfortably challenging" yourself, so adjust the weight accordingly. Finally, be sure to vary your routine every 2 to 3 weeks by choosing different machines for the different muscle groups. This will keep things fresh for your body—and your mind. A certified personal trainer can help you continually modify your routine, and many have backgrounds treating specific health conditions (so definitely see a pro in those cases).

BEGINNER ENERGIZE PROGRAM

MONDAY FF: Perform aerobic activity (e.g., steady swim) for 45 minutes in Zone 1. **TS:** Perform aerobic activity (e.g., moderate jog or swim) for 30 minutes.

TUESDAY FF: 30 minutes strength work; **TS:** 20 minutes strength work

WEDNESDAY: OFF

THURSDAY FF: 30 minutes aerobic exercise, Zone 2, and 20 minutes strength work; **TS:** 20 minutes aerobic exercise and 15 minutes strength work

FRIDAY FF: 45 minutes aerobic exercise, Zone 2; **TS:** 20 minutes aerobic exercise

SATURDAY: OFF

SUNDAY FF: 45 minutes aerobic exercise, Zone 1; **TS:** 20 minutes aerobic exercise

MONDAY: OFF

TUESDAY: OFF

WEDNESDAY FF: 60 minutes aerobic exercise, Zone 1; **TS:** 30 minutes aerobic exercise

THURSDAY: OFF

FRIDAY FF: 60 minutes aerobic exercise, Zone 1; **TS:** 30 minutes aerobic exercise

SATURDAY FF: 45 minutes strength work; **TS:** 20 minutes strength work

SUNDAY: OFF

BEGINNER CHALLENGE PROGRAM

MONDAY FF: Perform aerobic activity (e.g., steady swim) for 45 minutes in Zone 1. **TS:** Perform aerobic activity (e.g., moderate jog or swim) for 30 minutes.

TUESDAY FF: 40 minutes strength work; **TS:** 30 minutes strength work

WEDNESDAY: OFF

THURSDAY FF: 45 minutes aerobic exercise, Zone 2, and 20 minutes strength work; **TS:** 30 minutes aerobic exercise and 15 minutes strength work

FRIDAY FF: 60 minutes aerobic exercise, Zone 2; **TS:** 30 minutes aerobic exercise

SATURDAY: OFF

SUNDAY FF: 45 minutes aerobic exercise, Zone 1; **TS:** 20 minutes aerobic exercise

MONDAY: OFF

TUESDAY: OFF

WEDNESDAY FF: 60 minutes aerobic exercise, Zone 1; **TS:** 30 minutes aerobic exercise

THURSDAY: OFF

FRIDAY FF: 75 minutes aerobic exercise, Zone 1; **TS:** 30 minutes aerobic exercise

SATURDAY FF: 45 minutes strength work; **TS:** 20 minutes strength work

SUNDAY: OFF

INTERMEDIATE ENERGIZE PROGRAM

MONDAY FF: Perform aerobic exercise (e.g., steady run) for 60 minutes in Training Zone 1. **TS:** Perform aerobic exercise (e.g., moderate jog or swim) for 30 minutes.

TUESDAY FF: 45 minutes strength work; **TS:** 20 minutes strength work

WEDNESDAY: OFF

THURSDAY FF: 60 minutes aerobic exercise, Zone 2, and 30 minutes strength work; **TS:** 30 minutes aerobic exercise and 15 minutes strength work

FRIDAY: OFF

SATURDAY: OFF

SUNDAY FF: 75 minutes aerobic exercise, Zone 1; **TS:** 30 minutes aerobic exercise

MONDAY: OFF

TUESDAY FF: 60 minutes aerobic exercise, Zone 2, and 45 minutes strength work; **TS:** 30 minutes aerobic training and 20 minutes strength work

WEDNESDAY FF: 60 minutes aerobic exercise, Zone 1; **TS:** 30 minutes aerobic exercise, Zone 1

THURSDAY: OFF

FRIDAY FF: 90 minutes aerobic exercise: Zone 1; **TS:** 45 minutes aerobic exercise

SATURDAY FF: 45 minutes strength work; **TS:** 20 minutes strength work

SUNDAY: OFF

INTERMEDIATE CHALLENGE PROGRAM

MONDAY FF: Perform aerobic exercise (e.g., steady run) for 60 minutes in Training Zone 1. **TS:** Perform aerobic exercise (e.g., moderate jog or swim) for 30 minutes.

TUESDAY FF: 45 minutes strength work; **TS:** 20 minutes strength work

WEDNESDAY: OFF

THURSDAY FF: 75 minutes aerobic exercise, Zone 2, and 30 minutes strength work; **TS:** 30 minutes aerobic exercise and 15 minutes strength work

FRIDAY: OFF

SATURDAY: OFF

SUNDAY FF: 90 minutes aerobic exercise, Zone 1; **TS:** 30 minutes aerobic exercise

MONDAY: OFF

TUESDAY FF: 60 minutes aerobic exercise, Zone 2, and 45 minutes strength work; **TS:** 30 minutes aerobic training and 20 minutes strength work

WEDNESDAY FF: 75 minutes aerobic exercise, Zone 1; **TS:** 30 minutes aerobic exercise, Zone 1

THURSDAY: OFF

FRIDAY FF: 90 minutes aerobic exercise: Zone 1; **TS:** 45 minutes aerobic exercise

SATURDAY FF: 45 minutes strength work; **TS:** 20 minutes strength work

SUNDAY: OFF

ADVANCED ENERGIZE PROGRAM

MONDAY FF: Perform aerobic exercise (e.g., steady run) for 75 minutes in Zone 1. **TS:** Perform sport-specific exercise (e.g., moderate jog or swim) for 30 minutes.

TUESDAY FF: 60 minutes strength work; **TS:** 30 minutes strength work

WEDNESDAY: OFF

THURSDAY: OFF

FRIDAY FF: 75 minutes aerobic exercise, Zone 2; **TS:** 30 minutes aerobic exercise

SATURDAY: OFF

SUNDAY FF: 90 minutes aerobic exercise, Zone 1; **TS:** 30 minutes aerobic exercise

MONDAY: OFF

TUESDAY FF: 75 minutes aerobic exercise, Zone 2, and 45 minutes strength work; **TS:** 30 minutes aerobic exercise and 20 minutes strength work

WEDNESDAY: OFF

THURSDAY: OFF

FRIDAY FF: 2 hours aerobic exercise, Zone 1; **TS:** 45 minutes aerobic exercise

SATURDAY FF: 75 minutes strength work; **TS:** 30 minutes strength work

SUNDAY: OFF

ADVANCED CHALLENGE PROGRAM

MONDAY FF: Perform aerobic exercise (e.g., steady run) for 75 minutes in Zone 1. **TS:** Perform sport-specific exercise (e.g., moderate jog or swim) for 30 minutes.

TUESDAY FF: 60 minutes strength work; **TS:** 30 minutes strength work

WEDNESDAY: OFF

THURSDAY: OFF

FRIDAY FF: 90 minutes aerobic exercise, Zone 2; **TS:** 30 minutes aerobic exercise

SATURDAY: OFF

SUNDAY FF: 2 hours aerobic exercise, Zone 1 (60 minutes in the morning; 60 minutes in the evening); **TS:** 45 minutes aerobic exercise

MONDAY: OFF

TUESDAY FF: 75 minutes aerobic exercise, Zone 2, and 45 minutes strength work; **TS:** 30 minutes aerobic exercise and 20 minutes strength work

WEDNESDAY: OFF

THURSDAY: OFF

FRIDAY FF: 2 hours aerobic exercise, Zone 1 (60 minutes in the morning; 60 minutes in the evening); **TS:** 45 minutes aerobic exercise

SATURDAY FF: 75 minutes strength work; **TS:** 30 minutes strength work

SUNDAY: OFF

THE STRETCHES

As previously noted, it's important to stretch your muscles after each and every exercise session. Here's a sampling of some of my favorite flexibility boosters for pretty much all the major muscle groups you'll work in any given total-body workout. Combined, they can be done for a few minutes at the end of each exercise session—or they can be done several times each for a soothing, relaxing, stand-alone stretch workout (in which case, you'll want to include a 5-minute aerobic warmup and a 5-minute cardio cooldown).

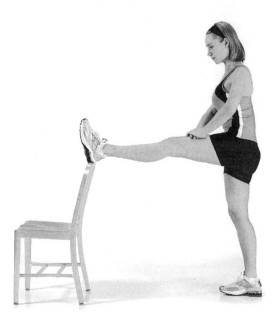

Standing Hamstrings Stretch

Place the heel of one foot on a chair or bench at about waist height. Keeping your back straight, bend at the waist and press down with your hand on your upper thigh, just above your knee. Be sure to keep your hips facing forward, not turned, with your toes pointing straight up and your knee soft (not locked). You should feel a good stretch along the back of your upper thigh. Hold for 3 to 5 seconds, then repeat 6 to 8 times, deepening the stretch with each repetition. Repeat with the other leg.

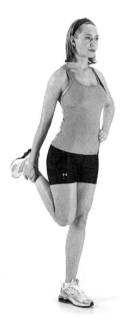

Standing Quad Stretch

Stand with your feet slightly apart. Keeping your thighs still and your knees slightly apart but next to each other, raise your lower left leg behind you, lifting the heel of your foot toward your butt. Grab the ankle of your left foot with your left hand, and gently pull your heel closer to your butt. If you have trouble keeping your balance, hold on to the back of a chair with your free hand. Hold for 2 to 3 seconds, then repeat 6 to 8 times, deepening the stretch with each repetition. Then do the stretch sequence on your right leg.

TheStretches

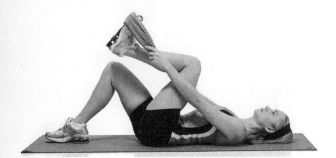

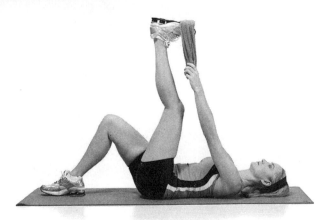

Lying Calf Stretch

Lie on your back on a carpeted floor or exercise mat. Raise one leg straight up with a soft knee (not locked), keeping the other leg bent with your foot flat on the floor. Flex the foot of the raised leg so your toes point toward your head. Wrap a rope, belt, or towel around the ball of your raised foot and gently pull your toes straight down to deepen the stretch. Hold for 3 seconds, then repeat 6 to 8 times, deepening the stretch with each repetition. Repeat with the other leg.

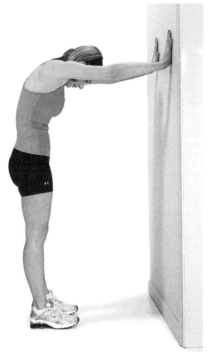

Upper-Back Stretch

Stand about 2 feet away from a wall, with your feet about hip-width apart and your toes pointing toward the wall. With straight arms, place the palms of your hands flat on the wall at about eye level. Lower your head so your ears are by your upper arms. Your back may arch slightly. Squeeze your shoulder blades together; you should feel a good stretch in the muscles of your upper back. Hold for 3 seconds, then repeat at least 6 times, deepening the stretch with each repetition.

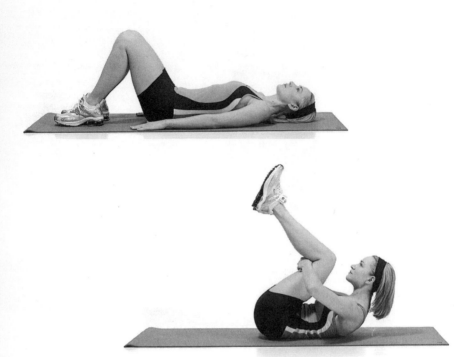

Lying Back Stretch

On a carpeted floor or exercise mat, lie flat on your back with your knees bent and your feet flat on the floor. Use your abdominal muscles to bring your knees toward your chest. Keep the small of your back pressed firmly into the floor while lifting your butt and hips slightly off the floor. When you can't bring your knees any closer to your chest on their own, wrap your arms or hands around the backs of your upper thighs and gently pull them deeper into your chest while exhaling fully.

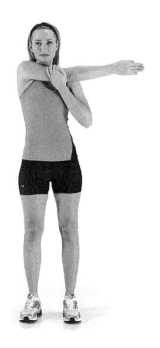

Shoulder Stretch

Stand with your feet shoulder-width apart, your arms down at your sides, and your abdominal muscles tucked in. Keeping your left arm straight, bring it up and across your chest toward your right shoulder as far as it will go. Then place your right hand on your upper left arm just above your elbow. Without twisting your upper body—in other words, keep your shoulders square—gently push your left arm toward your right shoulder a few inches more while exhaling. Hold for 2 to 3 seconds, and then drop your left arm down and shake it out. Repeat 6 to 8 times, then do the same with your right arm.

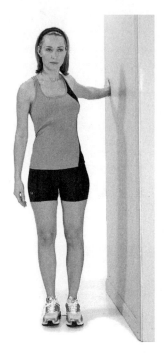

Chest Stretch

Stand next to a wall so that you're just a few inches away, with your arms
at your sides. Place one palm down on the wall straight behind you so
that your hand lines up with your shoulder. Keep your hips and shoulders squared and your free hand down at your side. Hold for 2 to 3 seconds, then repeat 6 to 8 times. Repeat the entire sequence with your other
arm.

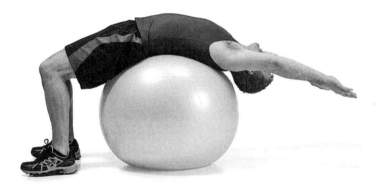

Ball Drape

Lie on your back on a stability ball, and drape yourself over the ball so that your pelvis opens up and you feel a good stretch in your abs. Keep your feet flat on the floor as you allow the pressure of the ball to run up through your hips and the small of your back. Your head and neck should fall down the back of the ball while you hold your arms outstretched in a natural position, with your fingertips grazing the floor for balance. Hold for 2 to 3 seconds, then repeat 6 to 8 times, deepening the stretch with each repetition.

TheStretches

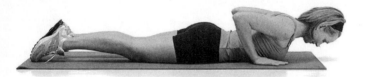

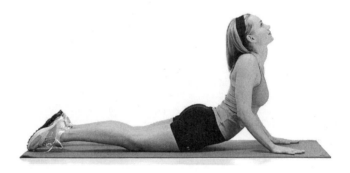

Cobra Pose

Lie facedown on a carpeted floor or exercise mat with your feet more than shoulder-width apart. It can help to "splay" your feet out a little to really open up your hips. Place your hands, palms down, on the mat directly under your shoulders. Now push up with your arms to lift your torso off the floor, making sure to keep your pelvis pressed into the floor. Keep your elbows bent, your shoulders relaxed (not shrugged up by your ears), and focus your gaze slightly higher than the horizon. Hold for 2 to 3 seconds, then repeat 6 to 8 times, deepening the stretch with each repetition.

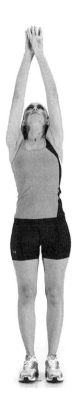

Overhead Stretch

Stand with your feet shoulder-width apart and reach both arms straight over your head, with your hands flat against one another and both palms facing forward. Fully extend your arms, point your fingers, and reach as high as you can straight up over your head, making your body as long as possible. Hold for 2 to 3 seconds, then relax. Repeat 6 to 8 times, deepening the stretch and elongating your body even more with each repetition.

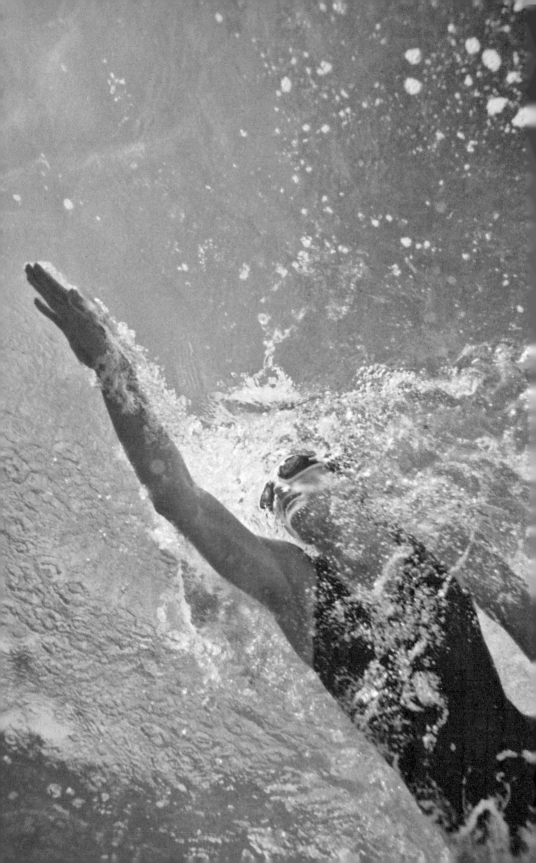

FOUR

The Next Level: Techniques for Maximum Results in Minimum Time

"We must use time as a tool, not as a crutch."
—**John F. Kennedy**

My assumption is that when you exercise, you'd like to get the biggest possible bang for your workout buck. After all, who wants to be consistently active only to get consistently average results? The goal-specific programs prescribed in Chapter 3 are designed to deliver significant and noticeable payoffs as efficiently and safely as possible. But there's no reason to stop there; whether you've already tried the workouts for one or more goals or you've made it to the advanced level and are ready to push yourself even further, there's always room for more variety and greater challenges in your exercise regimen. In fact, mixing things up as much as possible is essential if you want to continue to make progress, stay motivated, and stave off

< **97** >

boredom. And it needn't require a greater time commitment—just a little creativity.

There are so many different exercises, activities, and training techniques available to you, it would likely take a lifetime for you to tackle every possible option. In this chapter, I'm going to outline some of the most effective ways to get the maximum benefit from the time you spend working out. And while many of the techniques and concepts presented here are certainly challenging, research actually suggests that most of these methods can be safe and effective for beginners as well. So if you've got the go-ahead from your doctor and feel up to the task, let's explore some of the ways you can ensure the time you put into your workout program is not just well spent but a veritable bargain!

TIME-SAVING STRENGTH TECHNIQUES

Getting serious results from pumping iron doesn't necessarily mean you need to exercise like an oiled-up bodybuilder, nor that you'll wind up looking like one. In fact, research indicates that even a basic routine (as little as one set of 8 to 12 reps of 10 or 12 machine-based moves a couple of times a week) can lead to significant increases in muscle strength. Again, this doesn't mean a bulking, hulking physique (unless you're following the diet and exercise program of a bodybuilder and are genetically predisposed to accomplish that—and to you, I humbly apologize!), but rather a firm and lean body, efficient movement, the ability to easily lift anything from your kids to your groceries, healthy bones, and a revved metabolism, among many other things.

However, after about 4 months, your results may grind to a halt, also known as a strength plateau. At that point you've either got to put in more time (which usually means increasing the number of sets you do) or turn to high-intensity training techniques, which can save you time *and* pump up your results, according to prominent fitness researcher Wayne L. Westcott, PhD, of the South Shore YMCA in Quincy, Massachusetts. Here's a rundown of four of the most common high-intensity techniques and how they work. But note: Because these techniques require greater demands on your muscles, Dr. Westcott advises that you engage in them only once or twice a week for no more than 8 weeks followed by a more traditional routine for another 6 to 8 weeks; then return to the high-intensity drill again.

The**GoalDigger**Tip

Join the circuit.

Strength training is not typically associated with aerobic conditioning or a considerable calorie burn, but research has established that circuit training is one effective way to reap both strength and cardiovascular benefits. This kind of exercise has become particularly popular with women, as it's the cornerstone of programming at places like Curves. The great thing about circuit training is that you can accomplish quite a lot in a short period of time.

To perform a circuit, you simply move very quickly from one exercise to the next (ideally, no more than 30 seconds between moves). When it was originally developed at the University of Leeds in England, a circuit consisted of 9 to 12 exercise stations, and participants would work for 15 to 45 seconds (or perform about 8 to 20 reps of each strength move) at each station, using a resistance of 40 to 60 percent of their one-rep maximum. The exercises you perform in your own circuit routine can be as varied as you like, whether it's calisthenics or strength exercises (for instance, you might go from jumping jacks to squats to pushups, or from one Nautilus machine to the next). These days, a lot of people do a few minutes of aerobic exercise (like stepups or jogging in place) in between strength sets to further boost the cardiovascular benefits. The key is to move quickly through the circuit, resting only when you've completed all of the exercises. If you're pressed for time, just do one circuit (which could take as little as several minutes) and call it a day; otherwise, you can repeat the circuit as many times as your schedule allows.

Assisted Training

Have you ever seen a personal trainer helping a client complete the last few repetitions of an exercise at the gym and wondered how this could possibly be beneficial (aside from making clients think they're stronger than they actually are)? Chances are they were doing an assisted training technique: After working the muscle to fatigue, rather than stopping, resting, and then performing another set or more—which can obviously be time-consuming—the person doing the assisting simply helps during the lifting phase so the exerciser can eke out a few more reps, doing the lowering phase unassisted.

For instance, let's say you've completed 12 repetitions on a leg press machine and can't possibly do another. You then have a partner—perhaps a personal trainer or a workout buddy—help you press up the weight, but you lower it each time on your own till you reach fatigue again (generally in another two to four reps). In essence, you're pushing the target muscles as far as they can go twice in one extended set, rather than having to complete two (or more) full sets. According to Dr. Westcott's research, individuals who employ this training technique can boost their strength nearly 50 percent more than if they continue doing standard single-set exercises. In one study, participants who did standard sets of exercises on the seated leg curl and abdominal crunch machines could lift 20 more pounds after 8 weeks versus 29 more pounds for participants who did assisted training 4 weeks into the study.

Breakdown Training

Just as assisted training may seem like cheating but isn't, a similar principle plays into breakdown training. With this technique, rather than getting help

The**GoalDigger**Tip

Fail yourself!

If there's one thing people do wrong 9 times out of 10 when strength training, it's using the wrong amount of resistance. Whether your goal is to boost endurance (generally accomplished by performing more reps—15 or 20—with less weight) or strength (fewer reps—no more than 10 or 12—with more weight), you should still be fatiguing the target muscles by the final rep of each set. Since muscles adapt pretty quickly, you'll likely need to increase your weight by about 10 percent every few weeks or after 6 to 8 strength-training sessions. You should also push yourself to maintain your form and go through the full range of motion for those last few repetitions. By exerting yourself at this high level, your pituitary gland releases a substance known as growth hormone—a highly potent fat-burner, a health promoter, and the most anabolic (muscle building) substance known to humankind. Known as lifting to failure, this will help you make the most muscle gains in the least amount of time.

from someone else to extend your set, you get help in the form of a lighter weight. To try it out, after you've done as many reps of an exercise as you can, immediately reduce the weight by about 10 to 20 percent and perform a few more reps—again, fatiguing the muscle(s) you're targeting a second time. For example, maybe you're able to perform 12 biceps curls with 12-pound dumbbells to fatigue. At that point, put down the 12-pounders, pick up a set of 10-pound ones, and do as many additional reps as you can (most likely two to four more). Again, Dr. Westcott's research found significant strength gains for people who used this technique—they developed 40 percent more strength than people doing standard single sets over an 8-week period—and it beats the heck out of spending your time doing two or three full sets.

Preexhaustion Training

Perhaps you've heard of an advanced technique called supersetting, in which you do two exercises back-to-back with virtually no rest in between. Preexhaustion is one of the most results-driven types of supersets. Essentially, you begin with an isolation exercise that fatigues the target muscle, then further fatigue it with a new compound exercise that works the target muscle along with additional assisting muscles. The concept is somewhat similar to the aforementioned assisted and breakdown techniques in that you're continuing to work your target muscle(s) for a few more reps—and you push your muscles to exhaustion a second time with a little help, this time from surrounding muscles in the second of the two exercises. For instance, you might do 10 leg extensions with 100 pounds, followed by five leg presses with 200 pounds. In Dr. Westcott's research, the strength gained from utilizing this technique was identical to the gains made by doing two straight sets of the isolation exercise over the course of 6 weeks. Other benefits of doing this type of training rather than two sets of the same exercise: You recruit more muscle fibers and may even find it more mentally stimulating because of the variety, Dr. Westcott notes.

Slow Training

Okay, so you'd think that a technique called slow training would take more time, not less—but because you perform fewer reps per set (e.g., four to six repetitions per set, rather than eight to 12), it winds up being a wash. Sure, you're putting more time into each rep, but if you do the math, you end up with exactly the same time commitment. For example, with slow training, you might spend 14 seconds on each rep (10 seconds lifting, 4 seconds lowering) versus a standard 7 seconds on each rep (2 seconds lifting, 1-second pause, 4 seconds lowering). Holy cow! Twice as long?! Sure, until you consider you're doing half the number of reps—meaning a full set on the slow scale would take 56 to 84 seconds, and a full set on the standard scale would take, um, 56 to 84 seconds.

So if it takes the same amount of time as a standard set, why go slow? Several reasons: First, when you lift in a more controlled and deliberate manner, you activate more muscle fibers. Second, lifting a weight more slowly reduces momentum, and since momentum essentially unloads the muscle you're try-

The**GoalDigger**Tip

Refine your form.

Whether you're lifting weights or exercising aerobically, a flawless technique isn't just crucial for getting the most out of the your workout time, but will prevent injury to boot. If you're exercising at a gym, ask a trainer or staff member to show you how to use the machines correctly and check your form; a few minor adjustments and tweaks could make all the difference in your results. Some quick tips on weights:

- When performing a lift, focus on the specific muscle you're using. In other words, don't throw your back into your bench press by arching it and bouncing the weight off your chest. That works your back, not your chest.

- Go through your full range of motion to improve your flexibility.

- Don't hold your breath. For example, exhale during a 2-second lift and inhale on a 3-second recovery.

As far as aerobic equipment goes, one of the biggest mistakes people make is leaning on the handrails when using weight-bearing machines such as elliptical trainers, stairclimbers, and treadmills. Research shows that people often diminish their calorie burn by up to 20 percent when they do this. So if you're leaning on the rails and the readout on the machine says you burned 400 calories in your workout, you probably burned only

ing to load, reducing your speed provides more focused benefit to the muscle. Third, it's safer; you're reducing the amount of ballistic force, or high-speed/impact stress on the body, so you're reducing the risk of pain or injury. And finally—you gain more strength! According to Dr. Westcott's research, test subjects who engaged in slow training gained 50 percent more strength than those who performed their reps at a standard speed in a 6-to-8-week training period. This was true of both the "slow positive" technique (taking 10 seconds to lift and 4 to lower) and the "slow negative" technique (taking 4 seconds to lift and 10 to lower). Just note: You will likely use about 10 percent less weight than you normally would for slow positive training and about 5 percent less for slow negative. So there you have it: Who says being slow is a bad thing?

320—Doh! Here are some other form pointers for two of my favorite activities.

- **CYCLING: One of the most important things to focus on is the height of the saddle, says John Howard, former Olympian, seven-time National Cycling Champion, and founder of the Cycling School of Champions in San Diego. According to Howard, your saddle height should be set so your legs almost fully extend at the bottom of each pedal stroke. To check for correct leg extension, sit on your bike and pedal to the 12 o'clock and 6 o'clock positions. Your bottom leg (at 6 o'clock) should bend roughly 30 degrees at the knee. "Your hips should not rock back and forth when you pedal; that means your legs have to stretch too far to reach the bottom of the pedal stroke. If your hips rock, lower your saddle," Howard advises.**

- **RUNNING: Maintain an upright, balanced, and relaxed posture with hips, shoulders, and torso aligned. Lean forward slightly from the ankles, not the waist. Relax your shoulders so they're not up by your ears. Keep your arms, wrists, and hands relaxed and moving in a natural path, with your elbows bent about 90 degrees. Your arms should not cross the midline of your torso; keep them moving forward. Don't overstride; your foot should land underneath your knee easily with each stride, not out in front of your body.**

EFFICIENT AEROBIC EXERCISE

It's certainly true that if you devote more time to cardiovascular training, you'll get better results—whether your goal is to burn calories and lose weight, to boost your fitness, or to be faster or stronger in your sport of choice. The Centers for Disease Control and Prevention (CDC) recommends getting at least 30 minutes of moderate-intensity activity (which they qualify as "any activity that burns 3.5 to 7 calories per minute") 5 days a week *or* doing more vigorous-intensity activity (qualified as "any activity that burns more than 7 calories per minute") for at least 20 minutes 3 days a week. So how can you ensure that you make the most of your aerobic conditioning—meeting, if not exceeding, those recommendations while still having time for a life outside of exercise? Here are just a few ideas.

Cross-Training

Without a doubt, one of the biggest mistakes people tend to make when working out is marrying themselves to one kind of workout—and this can be particularly true of aerobic exercise. There's the guy who takes the same run through the same neighborhood 5 days a week, the woman who heads for the same Spinning or step aerobics or kickboxing class every chance she gets, the folks who do the same programs on elliptical machines or stationary bikes and practically zone out as they go through the motions. If any of that describes you too, no wonder you're not getting much out of your workouts! It's time to shake things up and take your aerobic exercise to the next level—and cross-training could be the answer.

I'm a triathlete, so obviously I'm going to be a big proponent of the multisport approach. But there really are so many compelling reasons for tackling more than one kind of cardio workout, whether it's within the same training session or the space of a week, month, or year. And while cross-training doesn't just apply to aerobic exercise (it can also mean you do a balanced program of strength, cardio, and stretching workouts), it's hugely beneficial to apply the principle to that aspect of your training.

For starters, it'll prevent you from suffering overuse injuries that are all too common among people who take their passion for one particular sport to an extreme. Let me give you an example: When your only form of exercise is running, you continually place the same kind of stress on the same body parts—and that can lead to everything from shin splints to stress fractures to knee problems to tendinitis. However, if you run on Monday, swim on Tuesday, cycle on Wednesday, and so on, your daily aerobic exercise isn't as hard on the body because it distributes the stress more evenly to your bones and muscles over the course of several days. That means less pain and fewer injuries.

From the previous example, you can also see how cross-training leads to more balanced fitness—a more comprehensive strengthening of your body. You won't just get great legs from running; you'll also get more defined arms and shoulders from swimming. And that's not just a bonus from an aesthetic standpoint. To make my point more painfully clear: Perhaps you're an avid hiker—it's the only kind of cardio activity you enjoy because you can breathe in the fresh air, take in the views, convene with nature, and so on. Then, one day, a good friend invites you to go mountain biking. You figure, "Great! I've been on

The**GoalDigger**Tip

Stretch between sets.

There is a way to boost your strength that doesn't involve lifting more weight or even doing additional reps in your resistance training routine; you simply need to stretch! According to studies by fitness researcher Wayne L. Westcott, PhD, of the South Shore YMCA in Quincy, Massachusetts, individuals who performed a static stretch for 20 seconds after lifting with that muscle actually increased their strength by 19.5 pounds, as opposed to a strength gain of 16.4 pounds in test participants who did not stretch between exercises. Need another reason to try this technique? It will also elongate and build your muscles concurrently, saving you time and increasing the efficiency of your workout.

those trails a million times." But within 5 minutes, you're completely winded and can't continue. How can this be? You don't cross-train, so your body is only conditioned to exercise in one way. If you explored a variety of aerobic activities on a regular basis, you could have avoided this morbidly embarrassing moment.

Meanwhile, by mixing up your activities, you keep your body and muscles and cardiovascular system guessing—helping to stave off the dreaded fitness plateau that plagues those individuals who get stuck in a cardio rut. Cross-training also keeps your mind guessing—you stay motivated and never get bored because you're always changing things up from one day to

The**GoalDigger**Tip:

Challenge your balance.

No doubt you've seen a lot of equipment that looks more like toys than training tools laying around the gym. Perhaps you've even discovered how fun and effective these things can be. From stability balls to BOSU Balance Trainers, Reebok Core Boards to wobble boards, foam blocks to air-filled discs, equipment that challenges your balance is all the rage in the fitness world today (heck, even doing a lunge on a couch cushion could be considered a move worthy of exercise trendoids). Why? It's an easy way to boost the benefits of just about any resistance exercise you can imagine. When you throw a balance challenge into the mix, your body has to recruit a whole host of stabilizing muscles above and beyond the ones you're targeting—especially the all-important core muscles (primarily your abdominals and spine extensors).

But balance tools aren't just reserved for resistance training. Cardio workouts can also incorporate a balance challenge, leading to a higher calorie burn and the same sort of additional muscle recruitment. That's the logic behind cardio classes that use the Reebok Core Board. "The board has an axis around which the board rotates, forcing your core to poten-

the next. And when your muscles and mind are fresh, you tend to exert more effort—which equals better results from the time you devote to each workout. Bottom line: "Cross-training will improve your overall fitness and, over an extended period of time, may ultimately lead to improved performance," says the American Council on Exercise.

Interval Training

Obviously, the more intense you make your aerobic exercise, the more you'll boost your endurance and performance, the greater the calorie burn, and so on. But here's the rub: Maintaining too challenging a pace won't just put you at risk for injury—it's difficult to keep it up for too lengthy a duration and can make exercise feel more painful and punishing than pleasurable. That's why interval training is so crucial to your cardiovascular program; it allows you to push yourself, but for a more manageable period of time—so you reap all the benefits of working harder without all the drawbacks.

tially react along all three planes of motion at once," says Annette Lang, Reebok University Master Trainer based in New York City. Think about doing something like a step aerobics workout (stepups, lunges back off the board, knee raises, leg lifts, and so on); now take that workout onto a core board instead of a traditional step and you've kicked the workout up a notch.

Here's a series of moves Lang recommends. Alternate toe taps by lying with your upper back on the board. Exhale, pull your abs in, then lift both legs, starting with your knees and hips bent 90 degrees. Lower your right toes to the floor, tap, then lift back up, and repeat with your left toes. Next, do pushups, placing one palm on each end of the board. After each pushup, rotate the board to the left and to the right, then do another pushup. Or try standing rotations: Stand on the board with your feet a little more than hip-width apart. Engage your core muscles, then rotate the board and your entire body to the left and then to the right. Your whole body should move at the same time as the board. Try these moves, and I guarantee you'll feel your muscles and cardiovascular system working harder than ever.

As you know from the Training Zone 2 cardio programs presented in Chapter 3, intervals involve alternating a more challenging bout of exercise with a less challenging bout of recovery. There are so many variations on the theme, depending upon your activity and what you feel up for trying. If you're working out on cardio equipment, for instance, you might increase the incline, resistance, and/or speed for anywhere from 30 seconds to several minutes, then spend a similar amount of time recovering by reducing the incline, resistance, and/or speed. Or, if you generally walk or bike on level terrain at the same moderate pace around your neighborhood, you might head for a hillier area, so the intense intervals are determined by how many times you climb. Or you could simply pick up the pace every few minutes until you can't keep it up, then slow down for a few minutes and repeat. Your options are as limitless as your imagination when it comes to the ways to interval train.

But now for the disclaimer: While intervals are a tremendous way to

The**GoalDigger**Tip

Set yourself free.

Resistance machines might seem like they'd challenge your muscles more than dinky little dumbbells, given the sheer size of the weights, but if you really want to build comprehensive strength, step away from those behemoths. Fact is, you can generally work more muscles in less time with free weights—and even body weight—plus build greater functional strength (the kind you use in your day-to-day movements). Why? The bodybuilding machines tend to isolate muscles and help keep you in place, while free weights and body weight-only moves require you to recruit more stabilizing muscles to maintain proper form and your balance. (And how often as you go about your day do you find yourself mimicking a move like a hamstrings curl as opposed to, say, a squat?) It's not that you shouldn't use machines at all—they definitely have their place, particularly for training your muscles to lift large quantities of weight. But if you mix things up—do crunches on the floor or on a stability ball rather than using an abdominal machine now and then, or go for lunges or squats in place of hamstrings curls—you'll have a better-rounded routine and likely see more impressive and even speedier results.

boost your cardiovascular fitness and calorie burn in minimal time, you generally shouldn't do intervals for more than 30 or 40 minutes in one work-out, since it can be stressful on your body. You should also limit yourself to two interval training sessions per week for low-impact activities like cycling, swimming, or elliptical exercise—and one session a week for higher-impact activities like running. Yes, that's how powerful interval training can be!

Everyday Activity

Nothing is more amusing to me than the person who tries to find a spot as close to the front door of the gym as possible—except maybe the person who drives to a running track or transports his bike to the location where he wants to ride. Sure, I understand it on one level, but on another I think it's just incongruous.

The fact is that there are a million ways to boost your cardiovascular fit-ness and burn extra calories from one moment to the next throughout your day—and they have nothing to do with dedicated aerobic "workouts." These are the everyday activities you perform, from running errands to cleaning the house to lugging your kids from one place to the next. Problem is, we live in a society that likes to take shortcuts. Advances in modern living—whether it's your car, robotic vacuum, or nanny—have robbed us of a lot of opportunities to move and, hence, reap the aerobic rewards.

That's why I suggest that on top of your regular aerobic training, you strive to maximize the amount of movement you get in everything you do. In fact, studies suggest that there's a strong correlation between getting about 10,000 steps a day (including your daily aerobic workout) and maintaining a healthy weight. To find out how many steps you're currently taking, buy a pedometer. (There are higher- and lower-end ones, but for our purposes, a simple little device like the New Lifestyles Digi-Walker—www.digiwalker.com—will run you only about $20 and should work fine.) If 10,000 steps seems like a lot, just wait till you strap on that pedometer and see how quickly they add up—and how you suddenly *want* to take the stairs instead of the elevator, to take the dog an extra block or two in the hopes that he'll relieve himself one more time before heading home, and so on. It's the stealthiest way ever to increase your fitness; you don't even realize you're putting in any extra time. (I know I sort of mocked it in the introduction to this book, but sneaking in an extra "everyday" activity can actually be beneficial; it's just not necessarily the *only* form of exercise you should get!)

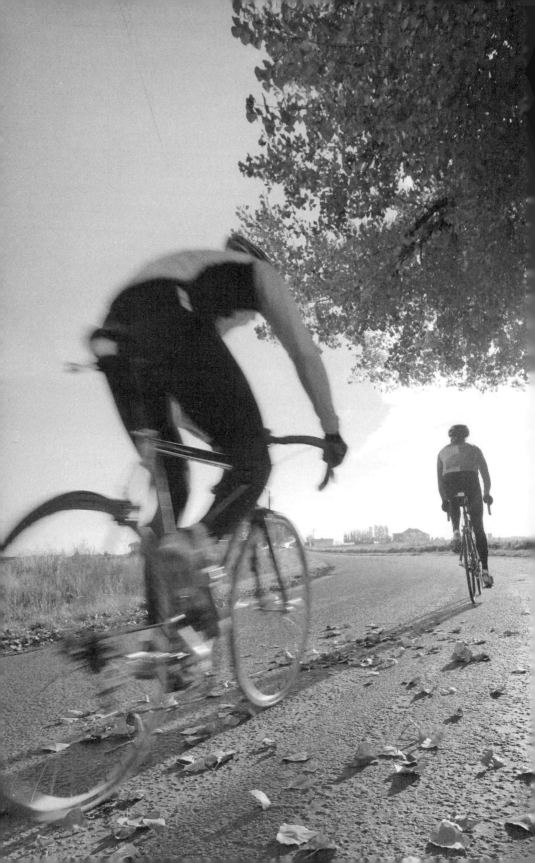

FIVE

Mind Games: Strengthen Your Psyche for Supreme Success

"What we think, we become."
—Buddha

As you probably know, physical activity can have a hugely positive impact on your mental health. Research consistently and conclusively establishes that exercise can relieve stress, increase energy, and combat depression and may even improve memory and stimulate learning, among many other benefits. "Your brain is a thinking organ that learns and grows by interacting with the world through perception and action," notes the Franklin Institute in Philadelphia. "Mental stimulation improves brain function and actually protects against cognitive decline, as does physical exercise."

Given all of this, we can certainly say that where the body goes, the mind follows. But the more ubiquitous expression is just the opposite: "Where the mind goes, the body follows." And while that could potentially be great

< 111 >

news, the mind, unfortunately, tends to have a way of checking out, steering us down the path of least resistance, deterring us from pursuing and accomplishing all those physical feats—particularly the more challenging ones—that would be so beneficial to us.

But while the mind sometimes insists upon standing in the way of a supremely active lifestyle (it's a common conundrum, even among avid exercisers and elite athletes), there are ways to train your brain and sculpt it into a finely honed tool that will work with your body to create your fittest self—and that's what this chapter is all about. First, I'm going to help you develop your ability to rid your mind of the distractions that tend to get in the way of workout success, in spite of your best intentions. Next, I'll talk about the many ways you can cultivate your confidence so there's no space for self-doubt—yet another success saboteur. Then I'll get into the various ways you can ignite your passion for being active and keep those mental fires stoked for good.

By the time you're done with this chapter, you'll be so stimulated, so fantastically inspired and intent upon reaching your goals, there will be virtually nothing standing in the way of you accomplishing whatever you set your sights on—and that doesn't just go for elevated fitness and a more active lifestyle, but practically anything in life.

IT'S ALL ABOUT FOCUS

We already discussed the importance of goal setting in Chapter 2, and I'm hoping that by now you've done some soul-searching and even filled out one or more of the Goal Digger logs that start on page 183. And while having a target, or several, can be immensely motivating, it still may not be enough to keep you focused. Why? In today's fast-paced world, most of us have become conditioned to multitask. Try as you may to concentrate on whatever requires your attention from one moment to the next, your thoughts probably have a tendency to wander and bounce around. If it's plaguing you to an extreme, you go see your doctor for attention deficit disorder—but on the whole, it's not a situation in need of medical attention; it's simply the by-product of a hectic life.

Let me give you an example: You've had a long, grueling day, and there's nothing you want more than to get a good night's sleep. You're so intent upon achieving some shut-eye that you think you might just doze off before your head even hits the pillow. But no sooner have you crawled beneath the sheets than you're wide awake, thinking about the laundry that needs to be done, your big presentation at work the next day, whether or not you should have screamed at your kids or dog or best friend or spouse for something that may or may not have been their fault. Suddenly, it's 3 o'clock in the morning and your goal—getting a good night's sleep—has been shot to hell.

In this situation—and so many others—a lack of focus can clearly be detrimental to your health. I'll share another potentially life-threatening experience of mine: While training off the coast of Morocco, in the midst of a 4-hour ride with a group of professional cyclists, I was having a tough time staying focused; I was pushing myself as hard as I could, but these pros were giving me a serious run for my money. Suddenly, my thoughts turned toward what they were doing. I was so consumed with how fast they were, wondering what riding techniques were propelling them, that I completely removed myself from my own performance. Just then, several cyclists behind me crashed and lurched off the road. A few had broken their legs, pelvises, and jaws. When I asked one of the riders who escaped the fray how the crash happened, he said, with tears in his eyes: "I caused the accident. I lost my focus. My mind was on catching the riders ahead of me, and my bike slid out from under me." Whoa. Serendipitous or what?

No matter what you're trying to accomplish, focus is clearly crucial—not only for staying safe and injury-free, but for boosting performance and allowing you to enjoy physical activity, not to mention life, more fully. While it can be tough to quiet your mind—and oftentimes the more you try to concentrate, the more scattered things become—there is hope. Here are some of the most tried-and-true ways to harness your hub and bend your brain in the direction you most want it to be.

Breathe

Sounds simple, I know. But there's science behind it. Breathing delivers oxygen to the various places it needs to go in the body—including the brain. If you didn't breathe, your body's internal oxygen levels would drop to the point where you would suffer brain damage and ultimately die. Meanwhile, research has shown that taking diaphragmatic breaths can reduce your blood pressure and heart rate and give you a stronger sense of self-control.

Try it now: Take three very deep breaths in through your nose and out through your mouth while relaxing all your muscles. If you don't find your mind becoming more settled and focused after three breaths, take several more until you do (or go on to the next tip). Now apply this to your workouts: When you're doing anything active, use this technique—particularly if you find you're zoning out and failing to concentrate. I guarantee you'll kick your performance up a notch almost instantly.

Meditate

For a lot of people, meditation is unbearably tough—particularly if your mind has a tendency to wander. For others, the practice borders on ridiculous: a New Age or psychospiritual cliché, with its pointless mind-quieting shtick. You don't have time to sit there and empty your head; you've got places to go, people to see! But whether you believe meditation to be impossible or inane—in fact, *particularly* if you believe either of those things—you probably need it more than you realize.

If you're still not convinced, consider this: Research has linked meditation to increased activity in the left prefrontal cortex—the part of the brain responsible for attention, decision making, and memory. In fact, one recent study conducted at Massachusetts General Hospital in Boston found that meditating daily for 40 minutes actually thickened the prefrontal cortex in the 20 test subjects! These people weren't Buddhist monks, as in previous studies, but regular, working-class Boston folks practicing a Western form of meditation known as mindfulness. One of the head researchers, Sara Lazar, PhD, told *Time* magazine in 2006: "We showed for the first time that you don't have to do it all day for similar results."

Additional studies have further established that you don't have to engage in the practice long-term; if you do it sporadically, its impact on the brain appears to be semipermanent. It also doesn't require that you sit cross-legged with incense burning all around you. There are as many ways to meditate as there are reasons for it and origins of it. Often its goal is to free the mind of all thoughts; other times it is to focus the mind on one thing, as well as to achieve a certain level of enlightenment—spiritual or otherwise.

For our purposes, I'm suggesting you meditate to sharpen your concentration, which is the basis of the following exercise: Begin by getting comfortable (sit wherever and however you like) in a dimly lit room or any area where distractions and noises are least likely to interrupt (turn off phones and anything else that might make a sound). Then begin the diaphragmatic breaths described in the previous tip. At this point, you can choose to either focus exclusively on your breathing—the inhale and the exhale, perhaps any sound you might make as you do so or simply the sensation that it creates—or select a word or mantra that seems least silly to you, whether it's *om* or *breathe* or *calm* or *peace* or *I am focused*. You can either speak this word or mantra in a low, controlled voice or simply think it over and over again until you find yourself calm and completely consumed with nothing but your breath, word, or mantra.

The more you practice this kind of meditation, the more you will train your brain to become focused in any given situation. You can apply that sense of calm and singularity of thought to your workouts and any other goals that require your undivided attention.

Go with the Flow

If the whole breathing and meditation thing has you flummoxed, maybe this will grab you: Mihaly Csikszentmihalyi, PhD, professor and former chairman of the department of psychology at the University of Chicago, has done extensive research on a mental state known as "flow." He presents this concept in the book *Creativity: Flow and the Psychology of Optimal Experience* as one of the most profound experiences a person can have. "Flow during exercise is an optimal psychological state characterized by an intense absorption, a clear sense of goals, and a feeling of letting go," says Dr. Csikszentmihalyi.

Similar to the meditative state, flow has been found by scientists to produce alpha waves in the brain that are associated with relaxation and intense focus. When achieved during exercise, this kind of awareness can also take your performance to the next level. Think of it this way: Musicians, artists, and athletes are able to achieve remarkable results when they focus all of their attention on the process because they are so deeply immersed in giving their best from one moment to the next. That's what you should be striving for in your workouts.

So how can you accomplish flow? It's sort of like taking meditation one step further—but this time, you must tune in to everything you're doing while in a more active state. Let me first give you an example of *not* exercising in flow: You head out for a hike in the midst of a frantic day. You don't warm up and immediately throw yourself into the motions, all the while thinking about everything *but* what your body is doing (your crappy day at the office, a vacation you're planning). As you complete the hike, you feel drained and more stressed than when you began—and you can't even remember a single moment of where you just were.

On the other hand, to achieve flow: You head out for a hike just as the sun is coming up. You breathe in the chill of the air and ease into a fluid warmup, seamlessly followed by a more intense climb. You take note of how the sun feels on your face, the smell of nature and the dust on the trail, the pace of your breath, the slight burn in your muscles on your ascent. You hit your stride, rhythmic and pure. By the time you're done, you feel refreshed, invigorated, and completely alive—and later you're able to recount every last detail of the experience to anyone who asks why you look so relaxed and content.

Bottom line, trite as it may sound: Flow is all about being present to every experience as you have it, making almost any moment—positive or negative—into something you can at least handle, if not thoroughly enjoy. If you can master this state of alertness, you won't just achieve greatness in your workouts, but will transform everyday experiences from all areas of your life into extraordinary ones.

Visualize

There's a running joke in certain publishing circles that people who buy exercise books and magazines hope that by merely reading about greater fitness, they will somehow achieve it—as if through osmosis. But those very readers may actually have the last laugh: There is some compelling scientific evidence that when you visualize yourself performing certain exercises, you actually become stronger—without even putting your body through the physical motions!

Specifically, in one study conducted at the Cleveland Clinic in Ohio, participants were divided into four groups: one that thought as hard as they could about strengthening the muscles of their little finger (doing a pinky flexion move), one that did the same thing for their biceps (doing an elbow flexion exercise), one that did nothing, and one that physically performed the pinky flexion. The training lasted for 12 weeks—15 minutes a day, 5 days a week. The incredible results: The people doing the mental pinky workout increased their finger abduction strength by 35 percent, and the mental biceps flexers augmented their elbow flexion strength by 13.5 percent, while the group that did nothing reaped no physical gains, and the physical training group increased finger abduction strength by 53 percent. The researchers concluded that mental workouts improve the brain's ability to send signals to the muscles, driving the muscles to a higher activation level and hence increasing strength. This doesn't mean you should simply think about exercising rather than putting your body through the motions—but it is an important lesson about the power of visualization.

The practice should be incorporated into your workouts as much as possible. Effective visualization involves all five senses: sight, sound, smell, touch, and taste. "In mental imagery, you attempt to reproduce the actual experience in your mind in as much detail as possible," says Jim Taylor, PhD, sports psychologist and author of *Prime Sport: Triumph of the Athlete Mind*. Similar to how rehearsals serve actors, visualization allows you to "practice" before the big performance, and the mental prep fortifies your ability to excel in the actual activity.

Here's how to do it: The night before an important workout or event, find a quiet place, close your eyes, relax your body, and picture yourself executing an impeccable performance. For 5 to 10 minutes, see yourself moving with strength, ease, and grace, and tune in to how it feels. Then, for a few minutes just before you engage in your activity, again fix your thoughts on what you're going to do physically. And finally, when you're actually performing, visualize how your muscles are working from one moment to the next—try to picture exactly how your body is executing the movements. When you do all of these things, centering your thoughts on the exercises—in the moment and outside of the moment—your abilities and the consequent body benefits stand to be significant.

Surprise Yourself

Another way to literally beef up your brain cells and improve focus: Stop going through the same old mundane motions. When you operate on autopilot, you simply don't have to think or concentrate as much as you would if you did things you weren't accustomed to doing on a regular basis. Believe it or not, there's an actual name for the latter: neurobics! It's essentially a series of ways you stimulate the five senses by doing unexpected things that shake up your usual routines. Based on research from leading neurobiology labs around the world—including that of Lawrence C. Katz, PhD, a professor of neurobiology at Duke University Medical Center—the practice of neurobics can help strengthen, preserve, and grow brain cells as you activate underutilized nerve pathways and connections.

Some ways you can practice this shock to the senses: Try doing an everyday task, like brushing your teeth, with your eyes closed. Or, don't speak during a meal with your family; instead, communicate only with visual cues. You can also combine sensory experiences, like smelling a favorite fragrance while listening to music or looking at a beautiful piece of art as you sculpt something out of clay. Other ways to awaken the mind: Take a different route to work, or practice using the hand you don't normally use to eat, write, or operate a computer mouse. Or, apply the principle to your fitness routine and try activities you've never attempted before (if something like yoga is on that list, you'll get at least a double benefit, since it involves so many other focus-friendly elements). When you throw yourself curveballs in these ways, you'll be amazed at how focused you become—during physical activity and in just about any other endeavor. (For more about neurobics—and proof that I'm not making it up—visit www.neurobics.com.)

Sleep

Simple fact: If you're not well rested, you can't focus on *anything*. Studies involving a "psychomotor vigilance task" show that sleep-deprived individuals just don't perform very well. The assessment test involves staring at an LCD screen and pressing a button as soon as an image pops up. People generally take 200 to 300 milliseconds to respond, but individuals who haven't slept enough take much longer—and sometimes actually miss the stimulus altogether. One recent study conducted at the University of Kentucky in Lexington also found that people who took a 40-minute nap improved their performance on such tests (after taking about an hour to wake up).

So how much sleep do you need? According to the National Sleep Foundation (NSF), the average adult should get 7 to 9 hours every night—but most people typically come in on the lower end of that scale (around 6.9 to 7.5 hours a night). There are plenty of things you can do to ensure some quality shut-eye. For starters, strive for a regular presleep routine (if you have a baby, you know how important this is for bedtime). This might involve doing something relaxing to wind down before bed—perhaps having a cup of (caffeine-free) tea, reading a magazine, or taking a bath. (Just make sure you don't take a very hot bath immediately before bed, as a cooler body temperature is associated with sleep onset, says the NSF.) It may also help to keep your room cool (ideally, 65° to 70°F) and as dark as possible (get room-darkening shades to block out light, if necessary). And it's important to maintain a fairly consistent sleeping and waking schedule—even on weekends when you might want to sleep in, says the NSF.

Meanwhile, avoid stimulating activities and environments—like watching upsetting images on television, doing work, and being exposed to bright lights—in the 2 or 3 hours prior to bed. Similarly, don't eat or drink too close to bedtime, and particularly avoid spicy foods, which can cause heartburn, as well as caffeinated and alcoholic beverages. "Although many people think of alcohol as a sedative, it actually disrupts sleep, causing nighttime awakenings," notes the NSF.

Finally, get rolling on those 14-Day Programs (if you haven't already)! "Exercising regularly makes it easier to fall asleep and contributes to sounder sleep," says the NSF. "However, exercising sporadically or right before going to bed will make falling asleep more difficult." That's because exercise may not only stimulate you but increase your body temperature for as long as 6 hours (and again, you want your temperature lower to induce sleep). The NSF suggests concluding exercise at least 3 hours before you go to bed.

Bottom line: A relaxed and well-rested body and mind are only going to improve your ability to focus, your workout performance, and, of course, your overall health. If that's not reason enough for you, consider this: A recent U.S. study, in which more than 70,000 women kept track of their weight and sleep patterns over the course of 16 years, found that women who get less than 5 hours of sleep a night tend to experience significant weight gain. Specifically, according to the researchers, the light sleepers were 32 percent more likely to have major weight gain—defined as an increase of 33 pounds or more—than women who slept for 7 hours a night. Now those are numbers that ought to put you to sleep!

YOU GOTTA HAVE FAITH

Once you've mastered the fine art of focus, you'll be able to concentrate 100 percent on what you want to accomplish. So what else do you need to ensure your success? A heaping dose of self-confidence. After all, believing in yourself is the key to productivity. There's even research to substantiate this. In a study sponsored by the National Institute on Aging, two groups of sedentary women were given a fitness test. Regardless of how they had actually performed on the test, one group was told they had scored in the highest fifth, while another group was told they'd scored in the bottom fifth. When the women subsequently worked out, the ones who'd been told they'd scored well reported feeling better and more energetic about the exercise than the women who were told they'd done poorly. Clearly, if you believe you can succeed, you more than likely will.

On the other hand, if you lack confidence, reaching your goals can become a challenge—if not downright impossible. And if you're like a lot of people attempting to achieve a higher level of fitness, self-doubt can creep in at the most inopportune moments. Even if you're bursting with buoyancy right now, it's important to plan for times when that might not be the case—whether it's in the face of adversity or simply manifests as a slight twinge of uncertainty about how to proceed. As Helen Keller once said, "Optimism is the faith that leads to achievement. Nothing can be done without hope and confidence." Whether that sunny disposition eludes you or not, it's always a good idea to have some self-assuredness exercises and strategies in your exercise arsenal. Here are some of my favorites.

Assess Yourself

Few things can shatter your confidence as quickly as hitting a snag in your program—whether you get injured, miss a workout session (or five—or five times that many!), or fall flat on your face in a step aerobics class. When these things happen, it's natural to question your abilities, to wonder if you're truly capable of accomplishing these lofty fitness goals you've set for yourself. That's when you need to do a quick reality check—to look at the situation as objectively as possible and regain your perspective and composure. Is your injury as bad as you think it is—and was it really a product of your abilities, or of circumstances beyond your control? Do you really lack the ability to stick with your workout program, or did you just get sidetracked? Are you honestly uncoordinated, or did you simply lose your focus (because you didn't pay close enough attention to the first section of this chapter!)? Looking at the situation from every angle—not just the most dire and negative one—will help you restore faith in yourself and realize you're capable of more than you might think.

From there, one of the most effective strategies you can employ is to instantly file the situation in a mental folder marked "past." After all, what's done is done, right? The ability to do this is the distinguishing quality of many a great champion. If you've been injured, you can set your sights on taking the necessary steps to heal and get back on track. Even if you haven't exercised in a month, you can look forward to heading out first thing tomorrow (or right now) and beginning anew with an invigorating workout. You can take that step class again tomorrow. Or forget about that old-school cardio workout—it's time to try kickboxing! It's all about moving forward. If you can't see the upside and keep going, then move on to the next tip in this chapter and find people who will show you the way.

Get Support

I'm sure you've heard the expression "you're your own worst critic"—and if you've heard it a lot in reference to yourself, well, nothing is going to be more valuable to your fitness success than other people who can knock some sense into you. Even if you don't have a tendency to come down a little too hard on yourself, having a support system in place is crucial for not just staying on your game but kicking serious butt. You simply can't afford *not* to surround yourself with people who will cheer you on when you feel like giving up, who will point out how far you've come when you're not sure you're doing enough, and who will tell you that you can do it when you lack belief in yourself.

According to sports psychologist Dariusz Nowicki, who works with Olympic athletes, people are 47 percent more motivated to exercise consistently when they involve their family and friends than when they go solo. "Studies have shown time and again that when people know others are watching them, they perform very differently than when they know they are alone," adds Nowicki in his book *Gold Medal Mental Workout.* He suggests that you tell everyone you know that you're going to accomplish something—like completing an athletic event—to create accountability that will drive you even further. "The more involved those around you become in your event, the higher your motivation becomes to do the daily workouts," he says. And the mere act of telling others you're going to do something might just make you believe it's completely doable!

Meanwhile, in one survey of 100 Olympic medalists, more than 75 percent said their support networks were the one thing most directly responsible for their Olympic medals. These are elite athletes who, in times of self-doubt and despair, are able to make it through trying times and conquer because of their support systems. I know this from firsthand experience as well: If it weren't for my parents, I seriously doubt I would have had the confidence to pursue, let alone stick with, my career as a triathlete in the early days. They always made me believe I could do it, even when I wasn't sure I could.

The**GoalDigger**Tip

Silence your inner critic.

If you suffer from low self-esteem or are constantly disparaging yourself, I firmly believe it's important to see yourself through the eyes of someone else. In doing so, you'll be able to quiet that negative inner voice and realize what's truly possible. The next time you're coming down on yourself, try this: Pretend your harsh words are being said in reference to someone you love (and hello—you should place yourself in such high esteem!). Then ask yourself if you'd let someone else say such berating things about the person for whom you care that deeply. Chances are you'll realize you're being unreasonable, and you'll stop that self-deprecating, self-defeating chatter.

You also stand to benefit from working out with training partners who share your goals and passions for fitness success. I could go on all day about how powerful it can be to exercise with others—but there are a few aspects that are crucial to making sure they boost your confidence. First, training partners should be at the same fitness level as you—or at least close to it. (If they're not as advanced as you, work out with them on occasion to boost your ego. If they're slightly more advanced than you, a few sessions together could inspire you to push yourself—but more than that might feed your self-doubt.) Second, they should be fun and full of positive energy. Third, they should have similar goals, or at least share your vision and approach to training. Fourth, they should be the kind of people who dwell more on the positives and bring up the negatives only in a constructive manner. If you train with individuals who have those qualities, I guarantee you'll be bursting with confidence over what's possible in your workout program and, truly, in every area of your life.

Anchor Aweigh

Sort of like the state of flow we discussed earlier, there is a mental technique known as anchoring—and it's a simple and well-established method for developing confidence. This time, though, you must steer your mind not just to the situation at hand but to prior successes (it's okay to reflect on the past when you're drawing upon positive experiences). "Anchoring involves focusing your attention, quieting your mind, drawing inspiration from past events in your life, and then bringing those feelings of confidence and optimism to the present moment," says Kate Hays, a Toronto psychologist and author of *Working It Out: Using Exercise in Psychotherapy*.

If you're having a tough time remembering any successes, think harder. Everyone accomplishes incredible things from one day to the next, whether they're conscious goals or not. In fact, from the time you're born, you're constantly succeeding, learning, and growing—whether you're starting to crawl or walk, studying for or acing a test, interviewing for or getting a job. The mere act of putting one foot in front of the other in pursuit of something is an accomplishment. In the context of your fitness, you've obviously experienced workouts that went fantastically well—whether you lifted more weight than you thought you could, stuck with your program for a full week or month, ran faster than ever before, or simply showed up for Spinning class. Whatever your past successes have been, think of at least one of them and remember how you did it. Then realize that if you could achieve your goal then, you can do it again now. That's what anchoring is all about.

Play Make-Believe

Acting is another technique that transforms you into a tower of confidence—and you don't have to live in Hollywood or be a Scientologist to master it. If you've ever watched a stellar athletic performance—like an Olympian in those final moments before victory—you've probably wondered how such people can look so thoroughly composed when they *must* be experiencing serious physical exhaustion, if not pain. Their secret is simple: They fake it. These top athletes are simply pretending that they feel fine, and consequently they actually *do*.

Research has also shown that pretending to feel positive emotions (forcing a smile when you're not feeling particularly happy, for instance) elicits profound physical changes in the body, including the reduction of the stress hormone cortisol. It's that same principle all over again: Where the body goes, the mind follows—and vice-versa. (Remember?) So if you think you can't possibly lift a particular amount of weight, pretend you can and see what happens (only if it's safe to do so, that is). If you're convinced that adding 10 more minutes to your walking workout will be the end of you, reframe that into an affirmative "I could keep this up for hours" and see just how far you're able to go. The more you tell yourself you can accomplish, the more feasible you act like it is, the greater your chances of success. It's just that simple.

WHERE'S THE FIRE?

Okay, so now that you've infused your fitness program with the requisite focus and confidence, chances are you're also feeling pretty excited about what's possible in your exercise—and in your life. You're likely beginning to feel the drive and desire to give it your all. It's pulsing through your veins. Now you just need to keep that passion ignited so you remain consistently inspired—for this is the key to truly achieving greatness.

Tour de France champion Lance Armstrong epitomizes what it means to use emotion to fuel higher levels of performance. If you've ever observed Lance in particularly strenuous stages of the Tour, you probably noticed how focused, inspired, positive, and passionate he was. He let his emotions well up inside of him and, much to the dismay of his competition, completely unfurled those emotions into the pedals of his bike. There are all kinds of ways you can do this in your own fitness program—even take your enthusiasm to greater heights. Here are just some of them.

Be an Idol Worshipper

I talk a lot about my heroes—especially my mom, who was the very first person to inspire me to take on something as monumentally challenging as a triathlon. Perhaps you have a close family member or friend you look up to. Maybe you're awed by the achievements of someone you've never met—someone you may have read about in a magazine or book, an athlete you've seen compete (like Lance Armstrong), or even an everyday person who did something incredible that you can't help but admire.

Whenever we observe what's possible in others, it helps us to realize what's possible within ourselves. So I suggest that anytime you witness an inspiring event or encounter an amazing person, you record the details—whether it's in a journal (like the one described in the next tip) or by clipping an article or photocopying a quote. Keep track of these motivational moments and look at them often—particularly when you're in need of a little friendly reminder regarding the vast potential for accomplishment out there.

Champion Yourself

Even more important than keeping track of the accomplishments of others is keeping an ongoing record of your own achievements. That way, if and when you hit a motivational snag, you can recall the passion you had when you first began and how rewarding your fitness quest has been—and can continue to be. I call this accounting of your achievements a success journal.

Keep your journal in your gym bag, and spend a few minutes after every workout writing down your successes. Or write at the end of the day, before bed. Pick a time when you'll be relaxed and excited about recording your accomplishments. Just remember: Because the purpose of this journal is to monitor everything that's going well in your program, you should only record your *positive* workout experiences and the lessons you've learned. That is, it's not a place to beat yourself up or keep track of what you haven't done. "Focusing on the positives rather than the negatives is more motivating and productive in the long run," says Susan Kleiner, RD, PhD, a sports nutritionist at High Performance Nutrition in Mercer Island, Washington. Remember, each accomplishment moves you closer to your goals, and that's worth celebrating.

As you journal, tune in to how you feel and what's making your training experience so special for you. You might also include a before photo of yourself (with an after photo placeholder) and anything else that motivates you—the aforementioned details about others who've inspired you, healthy recipes that fuel your workouts, and so on. Build it into a thick, rich, inspiring scrapbook that's deeply personal—and then tell me you don't renew your enthusiasm for your goals every time you look at it. (For a sample success journal page you can photocopy and fill out each day, see page 195.)

Compete for a Cause

Human beings have a tremendous capacity for gallantry. You read stories about this all the time: Regular people are called to extraordinary circumstances, and they rise to the challenge. Each of us has that fire within, but daily life doesn't often present us with the chances to feel heroic. That's why doing something active for a worthy cause can be so powerful. It taps right into our greatness, and believe me, the motivation is unlike anything you've ever experienced.

I suggest that at some point along the way to becoming your fittest self, you enter a race or participate in some form of activity benefiting a cause near and dear to your heart—something to which you have a deep emotional connection (perhaps you lost a loved one to a particular illness, you adore animals, or you want to help children in need). The more emotional you can make your daily exercise and the event itself, the more motivated you'll be—and the more the process will impassion you. A lot of people lose their excitement for exercise, at least temporarily, if it's not rewarding enough. Make it emotional, and you cannot be stopped. When you make your fitness mission bigger than yourself, a whole world of motivation opens up to you. It's really quite thrilling.

And talk about something worth putting in your success journal! Of the over 100 events I've done around the world, I've learned this one incontrovertible truth: The bigger the challenge you take on, the harder you work, and the greater or more emotional the cause, the more heroic you will feel. Physically, you reap all of the proven benefits that exercise gives: a sleeker, more beautiful physique; a disease-resistant body; and a longer life. Socially, by doing something active for charity, you inspire and elevate those around you—and you get the same from them. But psychologically, helping others is what I call a permanent imprint on your soul. The satisfaction gained by putting your body on the line to help others never leaves you. It's the "making a difference" part that fills your emotional cup. By doing something active for a worthy cause, you help others lead better lives while helping yourself look and feel your best. That's a winning combination. (To learn more about a very special cause that will help you live your best life while you empower others, please visit www.care.org/workout. If you do, you'll get me as your personal online coach!)

Give Yourself Props

Research has shown that people are a lot more likely to commit their time and energy to an activity when they can identify its benefits in advance—and there's something about a big payoff that keeps you excited about your accomplishments. That's why it's important to develop a massive rewards system for yourself, with mini-incentives along the way.

If you've ever worked for a company that was good enough to give you bonuses, you know how motivating a little acknowledgment can be (especially that of the monetary variety!). But you don't need someone else to acknowledge your hard work—you can do it yourself. I call this external motivation—rewards you promise to yourself after particularly successful workouts or other strides you make in achieving your fitness goals. For instance, when you've completed your first 14-Day Program, perhaps you'll get a massage. For each subsequent one you complete, you can promise yourself additional bonuses, from new workout gear or clothing to a trip to a fitness spa (maybe even one of the destinations that contributed recipes to this book; see Appendix 3).

My wife finds this strategy immensely inspiring. For example, she once set a goal of running every day for 2 weeks—and in exchange for this, she decided that *I* would buy her a new dress. I've never seen a woman so excited about running! She flew out the door each morning—practically pushing me out of the way, the promise of that new clothing keeping her fired up for 14 days straight. (At the end of 14 days, I fulfilled my end of the deal—and she looked outstanding in her new dress! The entire process was a blast.)

Beyond these rewards you give yourself, you should also be identifying exactly how your workouts are benefiting you. This can be physical ("Today's bike ride will burn a quarter pound of pure body fat" or "I'm going to take 20 seconds off my mile time"), emotional ("I get such a sense of accomplishment from my Spinning class"), or social ("I get to discuss last night's episode of *Desperate Housewives* with Kate on our hike!"). Focusing on these sorts of payoffs is often what motivates world-class athletes to train 7 hours a day for years on end. When you can clearly identify all the ways that you'll be rewarded for your workouts—both external and internal—you will rarely lack passion for your program.

So there you have it: When you exercise your mind as well as your body, you improve your chances of not only reaching your fitness goals, but surpassing them. And as exhaustive as this chapter has been in recommending the various ways you can flex your mental muscle, these techniques are just scratching the surface. As you practice these exercises, and as they combine with your physical activity to improve your brain function, I'm certain you'll come up with even more ways to marry the mind with the body and come out with successes beyond your wildest dreams.

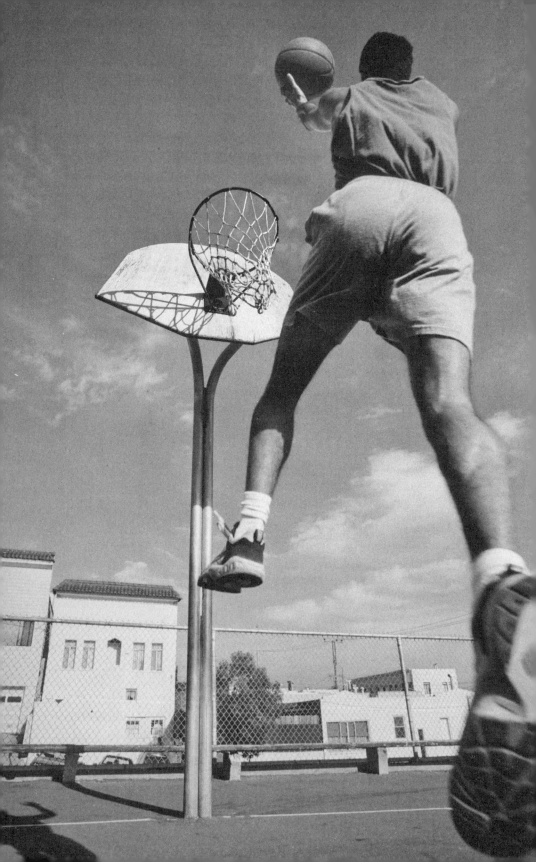

SIX

To Your Health: Preventing and Treating Injuries and Boosting Immunity

"The aim of the wise is not to secure pleasure but to avoid pain."
—Aristotle

While I don't entirely agree with Aristotle on the first part of this particular quote (it seems to me that pleasure is something we could all use more of and should strive for), I'm completely with him on the fact that steering clear of pain is one of the smartest things you can do, especially if you're trying to achieve a greater level of fitness and want to continue to do so for years to come. Unfortunately, most people tend to shrug off whatever it is that's ailing them—from seemingly minor headaches or illnesses to soreness in the back or various joints, like the knees and elbows. Admit it: How often have you felt a nagging pain somewhere, been coming down with a cold or worse, and simply popped a couple of pills (or dismissed the issue altogether) so you could get on with everything you had to do that day?

< 129 >

It's understandable. Most of us have full lives and don't feel like we can slow down for everyday ailments: "I can't let a little case of the sniffles or a migraine or [insert illness of choice] keep me from my important business trip or weight loss workout or family reunion or [insert immediately pressing obligation of your own]!" But what we fail to realize is that carrying on with our lives at the same harried pace, rather than giving our bodies the requisite rest and recovery when we're hurting (and even periodically when we're not), will only complicate the problems that plague us, often turning them into chronic issues and/or making them worse. We typically wait until we're literally immobilized by an injury or serious illness—until we have no choice but to stop and heal. And at that point, alarmist as this may sound, it may even be too late to resolve.

This is the last thing I want to see happen to anyone who's trying to achieve a greater level of fitness. That's why you must consult a doctor before embarking upon any new exercise program; it's why you should be getting medical treatment if you're experiencing any sort of aches, pains, or illnesses (even if they seem minor right now)—and it's why you should make injury prevention and optimum health your top priorities. You simply cannot unleash your inner athlete or accomplish much of *anything* in your exercise program—never mind take it to the next level—with a body that's experiencing even a modicum of misery.

Of course, there are a lot of things you can do—in your workouts and outside of them—to keep your body strong, injury free, and as healthy as possible. In this chapter, I'm going to outline many of those measures. I beg you to pay close attention to the advice contained herein—for in taking some of these steps, you'll inevitably enjoy greater fitness success now and in the long run.

DON'T GET HURT!

It is perhaps one of the greatest ironies in the world of exercise: You put your all into building a stronger, healthier body, and instead you wind up with a stress fracture or an anterior cruciate ligament (ACL) injury, you feel sore or sick or tired after a particularly grueling session—the list of potential problems goes on. When done properly, physical activity can make you feel better and actually help to ward off illness and injury. But *done properly* are the operative words here.

According to the most recent statistics from the Centers for Disease Control and Prevention (CDC), an estimated 4.3 million nonfatal sports- and recreation-related injuries are treated in U.S. hospital emergency rooms each year. "Exercise (e.g., weight lifting, aerobics, stretching, walking, jogging, and running) was the leading injury-related activity for women aged 20 years and older, and ranked among the top four types of injuries for men aged 20 years and older," according to the CDC. Meanwhile, a recent survey conducted by the department of family medicine at the University of Colorado at Denver estimated that even more Americans—to the tune of 6.7 million—report sports-related injuries each year, but that 2 million (nearly 30 percent) don't obtain health care for these injuries. That's a lot of people hobbling around with problems that either could have been prevented—or certainly should have been treated!

What can you do to ensure you're not just exercising safely enough that you avoid injuries, but that you actually build a body less prone to getting hurt as well? Beyond that, how can you care for injuries in a worst-case scenario? Here are some simple steps.

Be Well Equipped

You don't necessarily need a lot of gear to get a quality workout—but whatever equipment you do use should obviously fit well, be in good condition, and contribute to a safe and effective workout. For instance, you should wear clothes that don't chafe (including a supportive sports bra if you're a woman) and are weather appropriate (not too heavy in the heat, not too light in the winter), socks that keep your feet blister free, and shoes made for your chosen activity (see "Find Your Footing" on page 132).

Don't discount the need for protective equipment. You'll want to wear a helmet for cycling, for example, as well as for in-line skating, baseball, softball, hockey, skateboarding, and even skiing and snowboarding. If you play racket sports or basketball, you might want to look into protective eyewear such as shatterproof goggles. Knee and elbow pads are also a good idea for in-line skating, skateboarding, and snowboarding. Any protective equipment you get should have the approval of the specific organization that oversees your activity or equipment of choice—for example, the Hockey Equipment Certification Council (www.hecc.net) or the Protective Eyewear Certification Council (www.protecteyes.org)—or a safety certification from the Consumer Product Safety Commission (www.cpsc.gov).

Equipment that fits your body should be a major injury-prevention priority as well. If you're cycling, for instance, you'll need to find the right-size bike for your frame. "If your bike does not fit you, each time you turn the pedals, you are placing negative stress on your knees, hips, and back," says Warren Scott, MD, founder of Life Sport Medicine in Soquel, California. "That inevitably leads to pain and injury—so go to a bike shop and have them fit you properly on your bike." Meanwhile, a big mistake a lot of people make at the gym is not adjusting the machine settings—they just use whatever setting the last person used. But if you don't line your joints up with the axis of the machine, for example, this places stress on your joints and can lead to injury. Ask a staff member to help you figure out the right settings, or work with a personal trainer to ensure you're using the equipment correctly.

There are also a lot of safety and injury-prevention measures you can take in cardio classes that incorporate equipment. Case in point: If you're doing step aerobics, use a step of the appropriate height for your skill-set and abilities. That is, if you're a newbie, don't get ambitious and use four risers, copying the aerobics bunny who's been a permanent fixture at the front of the class for 10 years! I could go on all day about various gear and equipment specifications that warrant your attention, but the bottom line is that

TheGoalDiggerTip

Find your footing.
Worn-out or ill-fitting shoes can play a significant role in all kinds of physical problems—not just strains, sprains, and pains in your feet, but poor posture, impeded movement, and discomfort throughout the body, particularly the shins, knees, hips, and back. So make sure you replace your fitness shoes every 200 to 400 miles or after 4 to 8 months of training (whichever comes first), and buy them according to what kind of feet you have (that is, flat, high, or neutral arches). These two simple steps alone can help to prevent all kinds of issues.

Not sure what foot type you have? Here's an easy way to figure it out: Wet both feet and step on a brown paper bag or a hard, flat, dry surface. If you create a bricklike print showing almost the entire foot, with virtually no curve where the arch should be and no dry spot between your heel and the ball of your foot, you overpronate—your foot strikes on the outside of the heel and rolls inward excessively. Known as a flat arch, this can lead

you should use common sense and consult with the experts in your activity of choice—whether it's someone at a bike or running specialty shop or a staff member or class instructor at your gym—to check your gear for fit, safety, and experience-appropriate specifications.

Ease In, Ease Out

We already covered this in Chapter 3, but it bears repeating: Warming up and cooling down are crucial components of each and every workout you do, whether it's strength training, cardio, yoga, Pilates, playing a sport— really, *anything* that might qualify as physical activity. In fact, warming up for 10 minutes can reduce your risk of exercise-induced injuries by as much as 80 percent, according to the American College of Sports Medicine.

What kind of warmup is best? Stick with light aerobic activity that gradually raises your body temperature. This can be as simple as walking, marching in place, or simply performing the activity at a low intensity. This serves to literally warm your muscles so that they're more flexible and resilient— and because nerve messages travel faster at higher temperatures, your muscles will react more quickly, consequently reducing your risk of injury while

---

to arch strain and inner knee pain, as well as shin splints; shoes specifically designed for maximum motion control and stability can help. If you see a print of the ball and heel of your foot, with a slight outside border connecting the two and almost no print in the middle, you underpronate (or supinate), rolling outward (aka having a high arch). This makes you more susceptible to ankle sprains and stress fractures and requires a shoe with little or no motion control and more cushioning. If you see the ball and heel with a fairly wide band connecting the two and an inward curve where the arch is, you have a normal foot, or "neutral arch," and are less prone to problems, but generally want shoes with moderate motion control.

For more information about selecting the right kind of footwear for your activity of choice, as well as brand-specific shoe recommendations, visit the Web site for the American Academy of Podiatric Sports Medicine (AAPSM) in Bethesda, Maryland, at www.aapsm.org.

engaging in the more intense exercise that follows. Your muscles simply can't function safely or effectively when they're cold.

Similarly, perform about 10 minutes of light aerobic activity at the end of your workout, followed by stretches for all the muscles you've just worked. As noted in Chapter 3, this will gradually lower your blood pressure and heart rate so you don't wind up light-headed and dizzy, and it will boost your flexibility and help you recover from the training you've just done—all important for preventing injury.

Build Comprehensive Strength

It amazes me that some people still don't realize the importance of resistance exercise—they think it's something you only need to do if you want to bulk up and look "muscular." These people will sweat through cardio classes day in, day out, or do nothing but jog month after month, and they're convinced that's all that they need to keep their bodies strong and healthy. Not so. Strength training is arguably the most beneficial exercise there is, and it's an absolute must for preventing injuries—as well as for improving your performance in all those aerobic workouts you love so much. As 54-year-old university professor Jan Talbot—page 136—notes, an ACL injury sustained at age 34 stopped her from being able to run, hike, swim, and play soccer. It wasn't until she began weight training that she was able to return to running pain free, she says. It also boosted her fitness to the point where she was able to compete not only in marathons but triathlons.

Cardio simply won't strengthen your body effectively enough on its own. And did you know that if you don't strength-train at least twice a week, you'll lose approximately half a pound of lean muscle mass each year after the age of 30? That not only slows down your metabolism, but can contribute to poor posture and osteoporosis, among other things. Several studies have found that strength training can help lower blood pressure and LDL (bad) cholesterol levels, while raising HDL (good) cholesterol levels. It may also help decrease your risk for developing diabetes.

For the ultimate in injury prevention and optimum performance, your goal shouldn't just be to develop sheer strength. As I mentioned in Chapter 4, it's important to incorporate multimuscle exercises—like those you perform with free weights or your own body weight—into your program. This kind of "functional" training improves the kind of muscle strength, endurance, and coordination you use as you go about your everyday life. That means you'll be less likely to hurt yourself while exercising and doing pretty much anything—from lifting groceries to bending down to walking around, even getting up off the couch. Functional exercises also help promote joint stability and muscular balance—a good thing, since most soft-tissue injuries are caused by imbalances rather than weaknesses.

Focus on Form

As discussed in Chapter 4, paying attention to your exercise technique—no matter what kind of activity you're doing—will not only help you to achieve faster, more impressive results, but decrease the chances that you'll hurt yourself. For example, an excessively high vertical bounce when running can cause knee pain or injury because you place too much impact stress on your body each time you land (this type of injury is so common, it's actually called runner's knee and is characterized by pain around or under the kneecap at the front or side of the knee).

The pointers I offered in Chapter 4 regarding proper form when strength-training, working out on cardio machines, cycling, and running all apply when it comes to preventing injury, as well as boosting your payoffs. Other general exercise principles to keep in mind, according to the National Institute of Arthritis and Musculoskeletal and Skin Diseases (NIAMS): Avoid bending your knees past 90 degrees when doing squats, and land with your knees bent when doing jumping or bounding exercises.

There are so many potential ways to perform exercises incorrectly, it would also benefit you to seek the advice of an athletic coach, a personal trainer, or a group exercise instructor if you're not sure that you're using proper form—particularly if you find that you're experiencing strains, aches, or pains (beyond what would be considered normal) in your joints, muscles, or tendons while performing a particular activity. In that case, you should also consult a physician, as you may be in need of medical attention. (Additional information about finding an appropriate expert for your specific ailment is covered later in this chapter.)

Be Flexible

If you're like most athletes seeking to get more out of workouts, you've no doubt heard all kinds of information about stretching—and chances are a

University Professor Overcomes Injury, Competes in Triathlons

Throughout her 20s and early 30s, 54-year-old chemical engineering professor Jan Talbot of San Diego was the quintessential everyday athlete. She ran three times a week for 30 to 45 minutes and hiked, swam, and played soccer whenever she could. But during a game of soccer with undergraduate students in 1986, she ruptured an anterior cruciate ligament (ACL). She had to have surgery, followed by physical therapy for several months—but even after a year, it was painful to engage in the activities she loved, particularly running.

This was a wake-up call of sorts for Talbot. She realized she needed a well-rounded routine that incorporated more than just cardiovascular exercise— and that rest was crucial as well. In 1996, she started weight training. The resistance exercise helped her get to the point where she was not only able to run again—pain free—but was in better shape overall.

"Then, about 4 years ago, I started marathon training, and 2 years ago,

lot of the details are confusing if not downright contradictory. I've already discussed some of the benefits of stretching—to cool down and recover after workouts and, when done between resistance exercises, even boost strength gains, as touched upon in Chapter 4. Now let's talk about why there's so much uncertainty surrounding this seemingly simple aspect of a well-rounded routine, particularly regarding injury prevention.

The fact is, there are a lot of different ways to stretch your muscles. Researchers looking into a type known as static stretching found that it may do little, if anything, to prevent injury—and in some instances might actually make injury more likely! In one Australian study, more than 1,500 men were divided into two groups—one that performed 20-second stretches for 5 minutes prior to exercise and one that did not. The researchers found no significant difference in the number of injuries reported between the two groups. In another study, a group of college-age men performed a series of 17 stretches statically while another group did no stretching at all. The group that stretched actually experienced more soreness and produced higher levels of creatine kinase, an enzyme associated with muscle injury, than the nonstretching group.

triathlon training," Talbot says. Her current routine consists of an hour or two of exercise 6 days a week. "I now have goals each year; keep an exercise journal; and fit in running, biking, swimming, and weights," she says. If that weren't enough, she also hikes, backpacks, skis, and does yoga! But she stresses that rest is an important part of the plan as well.

Talbot also has had to surmount other obstacles to maintaining an active lifestyle. She says it's tough to juggle all her activities with a busy work and travel schedule—so she trains with a group known as the University of California San Diego Masters. "They keep me honest," she says. "If I'm not at the track, they call me at home to find out why I'm not there with them—and I better have a good excuse!"

While Talbot clearly enjoys being active, she also notes there's one noticeable payoff that helps her overcome any hurdles standing in the way of her workouts—and that's the way exercise helps her combat the aging process. "This morning an old marathon runner told me I could be 40 years old," Talbot recounts. "I happily reported I was 54, and I'm still smiling!"

Why might the likelihood of injury increase? Your muscles have a built-in "stretch reflex" that's engaged after either a rapid movement or 3 seconds in a stretched position. When statically stretched, your muscles protect themselves by contracting back to their normal range. If you keep trying to stretch the muscles while they're attempting to contract, you're in a tug-of-war that invites damage. Only a warm and relaxed muscle will allow itself to be stretched effectively. This is why experts no longer tell people to perform static stretches to warm up before exercise; as previously noted, you need to perform at least a few minutes of light aerobic exercise first—*then* you can do some static stretches if you want, or save them until the end of your workout, when your muscles are guaranteed to be warm.

The goal should be to improve your flexibility, rather than to use stretches as a way to warm your muscles. "Think of stretching as a workout unto itself," says Laguna Beach, California–based certified trainer Jay Blahnik, author of *Full-Body Flexibility*. "Just like resistance training, stretching places stress on the muscles, and the flexibility gains happen during the recovery period." The American Council on Exercise (ACE) in San Diego recommends that you devote at least 30 minutes to stretching, three times a week, for the sake of boosting flexibility—which, the council adds, can enhance movement, improve posture, and, yes, reduce your risk of injury while releasing muscle tension and soreness. "But even a mere 5 minutes of stretching at the end of an exercise session is better than nothing," ACE adds. "And all aerobic activity should be followed by a few minutes of stretching." So it really comes down to how you look at it and how you time it.

Of course, static stretches aren't your only option. Certain forms of yoga are excellent for boosting flexibility and have been shown to alleviate chronic pain (see "Say Yes to Yoga" on page 146). Many experts also believe that active-isolated stretching, or AIS, is one of the most promising ways to get the benefits of stretching while minimizing the risks. In AIS, you hold each stretch for just 2 to 3 seconds. Then you return to the starting position and relax. After resting for a few seconds, you ease into the stretch again, progressively warming and elongating the muscle in more of a "pumping action." In this way, AIS works with your physiology, not against it.

This is really the goal of stretching: to provide the means for muscle and tendon fibers to gradually relax and lengthen, thus allowing a full range of unencumbered movement. If you loosen your joints and elongate your muscles, your body will function more efficiently and with less pain. I know this from firsthand experience: Since I began AIS, my athletic performance has improved and a few minor injuries have gone away. For a detailed explanation of how to perform AIS, pick up a copy of *The Whartons' Stretch Book: Lifts for Over 55 Different Sports and Everyday Activities*, by Jim Wharton and Phil Wharton, which features a simple, 10-minute AIS routine you can do pretty much anywhere.

Bottom line: When done correctly, stretching is an essential and effective part of a well-rounded fitness routine and most likely will make your body more flexible, resilient, efficient—and less tight, sore, and prone to injury.

Be an Environmentalist

If you're planning to exercise outdoors, the weather is a factor you simply can't ignore. I'm not suggesting that a little rain or snow or heat should stop you from working out altogether; you can take plenty of precautions to keep the conditions from taking a serious toll, and you always have the option of heading inside if the situation becomes too extreme. Whether it's cold or hot, you should wear sunscreen. Use a minimum SPF of 15, reapplying as necessary, suggests the American Cancer Society, which also notes that "waterproof" sunscreen will protect you for at least 80 minutes even when swimming or sweating—while "water-resistant" protection may last only 40 minutes. Also, have plenty of water on hand so you stay well hydrated (we'll cover hydration in more detail in Chapter 7).

In fiercely cold conditions, you're at risk of frostbite or hypothermia, so it's important to dress appropriately. Go with several thin layers of clothing to help you stay warm while preventing excessive sweating; keep your head, mouth, and hands well covered; and wear waterproof clothing and shoes if it's wet or rainy. "On windy days, the outer layer should be of wind-resistant and 'breathable' material; the innermost

The**GoalDigger**Tip

Play it safe.

Exercising outside comes with a unique set of risks, whether you're working out on the open road or in a more remote locale. Law enforcement agencies recommend you carry identification with you at all times, make sure someone knows where you're going (or exercise with a friend), don't wear headphones, and stay a safe distance away from vehicles when near traffic. (If running, go against traffic so you can see what's coming; if cycling, ride with traffic, obeying all applicable vehicular laws.) Carry enough change for a phone call, or, better yet, bring a cell phone with you.

should be a 'wicking' fabric," says the Road Runners Club of America. Be cognizant of both the temperature and the windchill factor; if you're moving quickly (as when skiing, running, cycling, or skating), you'll also be creating a windchill. "When the temperature is 10°F and the air is calm, skiing at 20 miles an hour creates a windchill of -9°F," says the Mayo Clinic. "If the temperature dips well below zero or the windchill is below -20°F, choose an indoor activity instead." Be aware of the signs of frostbite (including numbness and hard, pale, cold skin) and hypothermia (an extreme drop in body temperature characterized by shivering, loss of coordination, and fatigue); if you suspect either condition, get out of the cold and seek emergency care immediately, says the Mayo Clinic.

Exercising when temperatures soar can lead to heat exhaustion, heatstroke, and heat cramps. To minimize these risks, wear light, breathable clothing that wicks sweat away from your body. Try to exercise early in the morning or later in the day, when heat and humidity are less intense. Take your workouts inside when the humidity is above 70 percent and the temperature is above 70°F, suggests the American Heart Association (AHA)—or when the heat index is higher than 90, according to the National Weather Service. Signs of heat exhaustion include heavy sweating, cold or clammy skin, dizziness or fainting, a weak pulse, muscle cramps, and nausea or vomiting. Signs of heatstroke include warm, dry skin with no sweating; a rapid pulse; high fever; throbbing headaches; and nausea or vomiting. If you experience any of those symptoms, the AHA recommends drenching yourself with cold water and getting immediate medical attention.

Don't Push It

As I mentioned in Chapter 1, it's important to pay attention to how your body feels each time you begin your workout—and, really, throughout your exercise session. If you're feeling overly fatigued, achy, or sore after warming up or at any point (beyond what's normal for you while exercising), you must honor those physical messages and *not* keep going. A lot of injuries can be averted by simply listening to your body, whether you feel like something just isn't right in a particular muscle, your breathing is more labored than it should be, or you're simply out of sorts and not sure why.

I'm a big proponent of taking a day off when you're not feeling up to par, rather than being out of commission for several weeks because you didn't listen to your body and wound up getting hurt. "If you continue to exercise when injured, further damage can leave you laid up for weeks or months and may even affect you for years afterward," says the American Institute of Preventative Medicine. In other words, skipping a day or two won't slow your progress—but continuing when you're not sure you should just might!

Give It a Rest

Even if you're not feeling any warning signals that your body needs a break, you still need to take time off from exercise. In fact, doing so is a crucial part of your fitness program and something world-class athletes emphasize and prioritize as much as the time they spend training. Why? When you work out—be it running, biking, lifting weights—you break down a little muscle tissue. If you don't give that muscle a chance to rebuild, your body will remain in a perpetual state of disrepair. That's why after weeks or months of consistent exercise, you can feel "heavy-legged" or worn out during activity.

As a goal digger athlete, your instinctive approach to getting fit may be to take whatever time you have and squeeze in as much hard exercise as possible. But that's simply not the best way to do it. In fact—and it's ironic—one reason people fail to achieve their fitness, weight loss, or athletic goals is that they do too much, too soon, too often. As many experts will tell you, it's during periods of rest that you actually grow fitter; the workouts simply provide the catalyst for the change. Not only do your muscles repair themselves while you rest, but you get an emotional and mental break from training as well—important for preventing injuries *and* making progress.

This is why every program in Chapter 3 prescribes 5 days on and 2 days off each week. On these rest days, you should avoid any kind of stressful exercise. An easy swim or walk is okay, but limit anything that physically taxes you, no matter how psyched up to exercise you may be. This will help you to harness your energy and unleash it during the five workout days you have each week. Hot baths and massages are good alternatives to activity on your rest days; they speed up the recovery process by increasing bloodflow and relaxing your muscles (see "Make Time for Massage" and "Get into Hot Water" at right and on page 142, respectively).

So how much time off do you need? When it comes to strength training,

TheGoalDiggerTip

Make time for massage.

Here's a good excuse to splurge on a trip to the spa: Research suggests massage can help heal muscles, boost physical performance, *and* reduce injury risk—and a lot of world-class athletes actually get bodywork up to six times a week! While that may seem like a luxury you can't afford (anything involving the word *therapy* seems to involve skyrocketing hourly rates these days), some experts suggest you can't afford to go without it. "Years of improper stretching, driving, sitting, standing, walking, carrying groceries, talking on the telephone, and working at the computer all lead to pain, injury, and general discomfort," explains alternative medicine expert Andrew Weil, MD, author of the best-selling *8 Weeks to Optimum Health*. Maybe that's why some health insurance companies are beginning to cover the costs of massage, chiropractic, and physical therapy—and it could be worth your while to find a plan with such perks, then explore them all.

you should never work the same muscle groups on consecutive days. And while you can exercise aerobically almost every day, it's important to vary the intensity and impact from one day to the next. If you're doing hard intervals on Monday, try a steady-state workout at a slightly easier pace the next couple of days. If you're doing something high-impact like running one day, swimming, cycling, or a session on the elliptical machine would be a good choice the following day, placing less stress on your joints.

Similarly, don't push yourself through the same cardio class day after day. Research shows that you can sustain injuries by overdoing a lot of popular aerobic activities. For example, one study of kickboxing instructors and students found that 16 to 30 percent of those surveyed suffered injuries to their backs, knees, and ankles, and the frequency of injuries increased when exercisers were taking four or more classes a week. This is exactly why it's important to vary your intensity and impact from one day to the next—and to take a break altogether now and then.

The**GoalDigger**Tip

Get into hot water.

Few things can melt away the stresses of daily life and help you recover from a particularly challenging workout as efficiently and effectively as a soak in the tub. I had my first experience with the true (and extreme) benefits of this after competing in a triathlon in Japan, when my hosts insisted I partake of the region's "hot bath" tradition. Painful as the super-sweltering water was, I nodded and smiled as they gathered round to see how I was enjoying my tub time—and afterward, I discovered every last muscle in my body was more relaxed than ever before. Not only that, I was completely recovered from my triathlon by the next day—a personal best!

There's science behind a good, hot bath: It opens up your blood vessels, allowing fresh blood to enter your capillary beds and bringing in healing oxygen and nutrients to your tissues while flushing out the waste. Now for the fine print: Effective as this therapy is, proceed with caution, and never take a dip in temperatures exceeding 105°F. Of course, if you're pregnant, elderly, or suffering from any health condition including—but not limited to—diabetes or high blood pressure, seek the advice of a doctor before steeping yourself.

If you feel you simply can't take a day off, this could be a sign of a serious problem—particularly if you use exercise to burn off calories. Yes, there is a very real disorder known as compulsive exercise, or exercise bulimia. While research on the prevalence of the condition is scarce, a University of Notre Dame Eating Concerns Survey revealed that more than a third of the 1,000-plus women surveyed exercised in spite of injury or other medical problems. Exercise was the most common eating disorder-related behavior among respondents—far more widespread than dieting, fasting, purging, or taking diet pills or laxatives.

Signs that you may be overtraining include dehydration and electrolyte imbalances (if you're constantly thirsty or have a dry mouth), an elevated morning heart rate, and frequent headaches. You may also be preoccupied with working out or use physical activity to anesthetize emotional pain or feel worthwhile, and you may become depressed if and when you can't work out. Experts say that in the long run, overexercising can actually lead to bone fractures, bone loss, and even periodontal disease. Talk about a counterproductive workout practice! For more information about compulsive exercise, visit the National Eating Disorders Association Web site at www.edap.org.

HEAL THE HURT!

Even if you follow all the advice contained in the preceding portion of this chapter, and no matter how hard you try to avoid getting injured, sometimes it just happens. If this worst-case scenario befalls you, the NIAMS suggests you cease the activity immediately—as in, the moment you experience any sort of pain. Then, it's time to get help and start to heal. Here's how.

Enlist an Expert

If you've experienced a bona fide injury, the last thing you should do is try to take matters into your own hands. "Call a health professional if the injury causes severe pain, swelling, or numbness; you can't tolerate any weight on the area; and/or the pain or dull ache of an old injury is accompanied by increased swelling or joint abnormality or instability," advises the NIAMS. While you can begin by contacting your general or primary care physician, I suggest you do so only in order to get a referral to a proven sports injury expert so you can get a proper diagnosis and effective treatment.

Let me elaborate on this. Early in my career, I injured my lower back—not just impeding my athletic performance but diminishing my quality of life more than I ever imagined it could. For the next 2 years, I saw a slew of doctors who advised me to stretch—which I did at least 2 hours a day. Unfortunately, the stretching didn't help—it made matters worse. When I finally found my way to a sports specialist, he discovered (within a mere 20 minutes, I might add) that I had a chronic muscle tear and said I would need deep-tissue bodywork to realign the muscle fibers. Six months later, with the appropriate treatment, the injury was no more. Had I met this good doctor sooner, I would have saved myself hundreds of hours, thousands of dollars, and immeasurable amounts of pain.

Of course we count on doctors to know what they're doing—but they can't possibly be familiar with every last ailment a patient might experience. That's why my best advice is to do your homework and ask your general practitioner to refer you to an orthopedist or sports medicine doctor (a specialist in the diagnosis and treatment of problems with the musculoskeletal system, including your bones, joints, ligaments, tendons, muscles, and nerves). Look for a professional with specific skills and experience treating your exact type of pain or injury. If you hurt your elbow playing tennis, for instance, find someone who is familiar with that part of the body and the activity itself. The American Academy of Orthopaedic Surgeons (AAOS) Web site (www.aaos.org) has a decent "Find an Orthopaedist" search engine that may be helpful (if your own doctor isn't).

The**GoalDigger**Tip

Quell your cramps.

The everyday athlete, no matter what his or her fitness level, is bound to experience a muscle cramp now and then, either during or immediately after physical activity. The good news is that this is essentially a mild acute injury (though it may not feel like it at the time!), and, while it may be painful, you can probably prevent or even treat the problem yourself.

What causes these cramps? There are a number of theories—everything from electrolyte imbalances to inadequate conditioning to overexertion to fatigue to dehydration to stretching habits. The most recent research suggests muscle fatigue is to blame, says Liz Applegate, PhD, a nationally recognized expert on nutrition and performance and a faculty member of the nutrition department at the University of California, Davis. "Fatigue brings on a series of internal changes that cause the muscle to enter a state of enhanced excitability," she says. "Then the involved muscle suddenly shortens, resulting in a painful muscle cramp."

Be Diligent about Diagnosis

Sometimes figuring out what's wrong with you and how it should be treated is simple—other times, not so much. The more recent and specific your problem, the easier it may be to address. Generally known as acute injuries, these afflictions typically arise from incidents you can readily put your finger on: spraining your ankle or wrist during a fall or, if you're like me, hitting your head on the side of the pool during a poorly timed flip turn. Beyond things like sprains and concussions, acute injuries may include broken bones as well as muscle, tendon, and ligament tears.

Then there are the conundrums known as chronic injuries. This type of injury is trickier to diagnose because it's probably been plaguing you for a fairly long time, and you may not be sure exactly how it happened or why it's persisting. It could be an overuse injury such as tendinitis, shin splints, or plantar fasciitis (inflammation in the arch of the foot)—or an acute injury that was never resolved (like the muscle tear in my back). And remember my mention of hurting your elbow while playing tennis? "Most patients with tennis elbow are not active in racket sports," says the AAOS. "Most of the time, there is not a specific traumatic injury before symptoms

---

To stop cramps before they start, always warm up (there's that advice again!); increase your physical activity gradually (another reason to begin Chapter 3's 14-Day Programs at your experience-appropriate level); and drink enough fluids before, during, and after exercise (two 8-ounce glasses of water before your workout, 32 ounces every hour during exercise, and two more 8-ounce glasses afterward).

If you still fall victim to an exercise-induced muscle cramp, immediately try to relax the spasm by stretching the affected muscle. Then drink plenty of fluids (either water or an electrolyte-containing beverage like Gatorade), rest, and assess whether or not the cramping may be due to something like heat (see "Be an Environmentalist" on page 138 for precautionary measures and treatments when exercising in hot weather). If your cramps recur frequently, it's time to talk to your doctor.

The**GoalDigger**Tip

Say yes to yoga.

Nearly 30 percent of Americans suffer from chronic pain. If you're one of them, research suggests that relief could be just a sticky mat away. In a study conducted at Harbor UCLA Medical Center in Los Angeles, 18 men and women with persistent chronic pain attended three 90-minute Iyengar yoga classes three times a week for a month. (Iyengar is a specific type of yoga that focuses on breathing as well as developing strength, flexibility, and stability by gradually increasing how long you hold challenging poses.) By the end of the study, the participants— whose specific ailments included low back pain, carpal tunnel syndrome, migraines, dermatomyositis, hip and neck pain, and osteoarthritis—were using less pain medication and had reduced their anxiety levels and boosted their moods to boot. Lead researcher Sonia Gaur, MD, says a larger study is needed to determine whether yoga can actually *cure* chronic pain, but is certain it can help to alleviate it.

start. Many individuals with tennis elbow are involved in work or recreational activities that require repetitive and vigorous use of the forearm muscles"—like painting, raking, plumbing, and the ever-popular weaving! Since chronic injuries can be so complicated, it's that much more critical that you seek out an expert in sports medicine, approach the problem(s) holistically, and be unrelenting about getting the appropriate diagnosis and treatment. That due diligence is all down to you; it's not just prudent but imperative.

Mind Your Meds

Oftentimes the specialist you see for your injury will recommend medication as part of your healing plan, whether it's an over-the-counter nonsteroidal anti-inflammatory drug (NSAID), such as Tylenol or Advil, or a stronger prescription. Popping these pills can be a great way to relieve the pain, helping you to more comfortably put a proactive, long-term healing plan in place. But this is just a temporary quick fix—a Band-Aid, if you will—and will only mask the problem if you keep medicating long term.

Eventually, your doctor should take you off the drugs; they'll make it difficult to tell if the bodywork, physical therapy, or other treatments you're undergoing are working—or if you need to resort to something like surgery or steroid injections. The goal is to completely heal your injury, not hide it.

BOOST YOUR IMMUNITY

I don't need to tell you that there's a lot more to keeping your body operating at its peak, above and beyond doing the right kind of exercise—as covered extensively up to this point—and preventing (or treating) the injuries that such activity may cause. If you're truly going to unleash the athlete within, never to be lost again, you *must* protect and preserve your health, and that comes down to strengthening your immune system in every way possible. When your body's natural defenses are fortified, your chances of reaching every last one of your goals skyrocket ... but when your immune system is weak, you're a sitting duck, primed and ready for illness to attack.

Just about everything I've advised you to do throughout this book will help boost your health and immunity—from getting the right amount of exercise (being sedentary has been shown to impair the immune system, as has overexercising) to sleeping and meditating (both of which can reduce stress; see below for more regarding how stress harms immunity). You also need to eat a balanced, nutrient-rich diet, and there are plenty of strategies detailed in the next chapter to help you accomplish this.

But believe it or not, there are even *more* steps you can take—measures scientifically proven to help you ward off illness and protect you from the biological agents that might conspire against you, depleting your energy and preventing you from achieving your everyday athletic best. These strategies, while basic enough, are so simple—even surprising—that they tend to get overlooked. So I'm going to bash them over your head in the name of unfaltering fitness, once and for all. Think of them as the final pieces in your unstoppable, totally powered-up puzzle.

Squelch Stress

I've talked a lot about the importance of rest and relaxation, and here's yet another reason you should make R&R your raison d'être: Research has shown that chronic anxiety can weaken your immune system, making you more susceptible to illness. The science is simple enough: When you're stressed out, your body produces more cortisol and adrenaline—the hormones that shut down the immune response. This explains why people tend to catch colds or experience other infections when they're overbusy, overburdened, or otherwise overwhelmed. (And if that doesn't grab your attention, elevated levels of cortisol have been implicated in elevated levels of … belly fat!)

Stress can also have the opposite effect on your immune system, making it overactive, according to the Mayo Clinic: "The result is an increased risk of autoimmune diseases, in which your immune system attacks your body's own cells. Stress can also worsen the symptoms of autoimmune diseases. For example, stress is one of the triggers for the sporadic flare-ups of symptoms in lupus."

Of course, telling someone to relax when they're stressed is hardly helpful (so my apologies for beginning this section in such an annoying way). But there are ways you can keep anxiety in check—including, but not limited to, a lot of the mind games recommended in Chapter 5 (breathing, meditating, achieving flow and focus, and engaging in confidence-boosting exercises).

Siberian Stress-Buster

Playwright Jane Wagner once said: "Reality is the leading cause of stress amongst those in touch with it." Since we all live in reality—well, most of us anyway—we're likely to experience stress. And getting stressed out is hard to avoid. Recent medical studies indicate that a growing number of people are more stressed than ever. According to The National Institute of Mental Health, roughly one in three people suffers from moderate to severe stress on a daily basis. This can have grave and long-term effects on one's health.

You can help your body manage stress better by including, and excluding, certain foods. The quality of the food you eat in large part determines the quality of the life you live. First, strive to eat a balanced diet filled with fresh vegetables (organic if possible), lean meats (free range if possible), and quality fats found in extra virgin olive oil and fish such as wild salmon. The National Institutes of Health also offers this suggestion: Eliminate or reduce your intake of caffeine or other stimulants since they just make things

Beyond that, I recommend journaling and making lists, figuring out the source of your stress, and then putting an action plan in place for alleviating it. If you're overextended by a hectic schedule, find ways to delegate some responsibilities (at work or at home; have someone watch your kids a couple times a week, for example). If certain people in your life are making you angry or upset or miserable—often referred to as toxic relationships—do your best to limit interaction with these folks, if not sever ties with them completely.

For every stressful situation in which you find yourself, there is probably a solution. It just comes down to brainstorming ways to overcome or eliminate your anxiety-causing factors so they don't become ongoing issues. After all, a small amount of stress won't hurt your immune system and can often protect you, spurring you to action (known as the fight-or-flight response); some studies even show that short bursts of stress can improve immune

---

worse. (I know, this is a tough tip to put into action, but it's worth a try!)

You can also su pport your body's ability to fight stress by exploring herbal supplements. Now, let me start by saying that most nutritional supplements simply don't live up to their promises, but some do. There are a select few products that have been shown to help to manage and reduce stress. Siberian Eleuthero is one of the most promising—as it the most researched herb in the world. Siberian Eleuthero is known as an "adaptogen," a substance that helps the body better deal with stress. As with any herbal product, you want to look at potency. A product called Sibergin® is the world's leading high-potency Siberian Eleuthero. Used and prescribed by medical doctors, holistic practitioners, and athletic trainers in Europe and America, Siberian Eleuthero can be an effective adjunct to any health-enhancing or athletic training program. I've been taking this supplement off and on for almost a decade and it has worked wonders in helping me beat the stress from my athletic and media careers. It is manufactured by HealthAid America, a reliable and recognized leader in the natural supplement industry. HealthAid products are offered at health food stores across America. For more information, visit www.healthaidamerica.com or call (800) 320-5699.

system function. It's generally stress of the chronic and persistent variety that causes the body to shut down and struggle to recover.

Find Your Funny Bone

Have you ever noticed how you feel better when you enjoy a good laugh? Science has a very good explanation for this: According to researchers at Indiana State University, laughter actually increases natural killer (NK) cells—white blood cells that make up a major part of the immune system and defend the body against viruses and other pathogens. In this study, 33 healthy women were divided into two groups; one watched a funny video while the other watched a video about tourism. Blood tests taken before and after the experience revealed that the humor group had a significantly higher number of NK cells after watching the video than the boring-tourism group did (I guess travel is no laughing matter!).

"When you laugh, there are opium-like chemicals released by your brain," explains Michael Miller, MD, director for preventive cardiology at the University of Maryland Medical Center in Baltimore, who has also studied the effects of laughter. "These [chemicals] give you a feeling of well-being or even euphoria. We believe this causes you to relax and your blood vessels to dilate. Laughter lowers blood pressure and your pulse rate. My advice is to laugh heartily for at least 5 minutes a day. Try to see the funny side and take life less seriously."

Pollutant-Proof Your Pad

You're probably aware of the fact that the air pollution outside can harm your health—but here's something that might surprise you: Studies of human exposure to air pollutants conducted by the U.S. Environmental Protection Agency (EPA) have found that *indoor* levels of many pollutants can be three to five times higher (and in some cases over 100 times higher) than outdoor levels! That's quite a problem, given that people spend about 90 percent of their time indoors; in fact, the EPA ranks indoor air pollution among the top five environmental risks to public health.

There are a number of culprits responsible for these indoor issues. One has to do with housecleaning agents, paint, and other poisonous agents you may have sitting under your kitchen and/or bathroom sinks. Our bodies aren't equipped to neutralize the chemicals found in many of these products, and this places undue stress on our immune systems, increasing levels of fatigue and illness. Home-health experts suggest substituting natural products, such as Orange Glo furniture cleaner or WORX WindoZ glass cleaner, whenever possible. In the case of any toxic products you can't do without, keep them in a sealed box or banish them to a garage or basement—far away from your primary living spaces.

Another problem: gas stoves and appliances that release fumes into the air. Solar or electrical heating devices are better for the indoor environment. Experts recommend that if you do use gas appliances, the rooms in which they are contained are well ventilated. Since the by-product of burning any type of fuel is carbon monoxide (CO), the Consumer Product Safety Commission recommends that every home have at least one CO detector and that consumers have their furnaces, water heaters, and other fuel-burning appliances inspected yearly by a qualified professional.

Meanwhile, paraffin—a petroleum-based ingredient used to make candles as well as to soften your hands and feet during manicures and pedicures—is a known pollutant. Candles also release soot, and ones with metal wicks emit lead as well. If you must burn candles, use unscented, natural beeswax types—and skip those silky-soft hand-and-foot treatments at the spa.

Finally, tightly sealed buildings can trap pollutants indoors. Your body depends on a rich, clean supply of oxygen to function properly and maintain optimal health. Unfortunately, in an effort to conserve energy, most homes are equipped with airtight windows, heavily insulated walls, and even gaskets

The**GoalDigger**Tip

Kick butts.

I almost didn't include this advice, because my assumption is that if you're trying to take your fitness to greater heights, you should *certainly* be aware of the dangers of smoking, and cigarettes aren't even an issue for you. But just in case you need to be told (or some tobacco-toting friend of yours is leafing through this book): The simple fact is that smoking suppresses immune cells—hence the reason smokers are at risk for lung cancer and other respiratory diseases (and pretty much always seem to be hacking and unhealthy). The good news: Immune activity improves within just 30 days of quitting. So, if you are an oxymoron of the fitness world—a smoking exerciser—now's the time to kick the habit, once and for all ... and boost your immunity in just 1 month.

that seal up doors and windows. Although these advances are effective at holding in heat and keeping out cold, they also trap contaminated air inside your home. According to one study, people living in energy-efficient buildings were 50 percent more likely to contract upper respiratory diseases than people living in older, more ventilated homes!

I drive my wife crazy because I'm constantly opening all the windows in our home to bring in fresh air—but it's crucial to our overall health. So I suggest you do the same: Open your windows often to increase cross ventilation. Also, consider installing a high-efficiency particulate air (HEPA) filter in your home, which removes particles in the air by forcing it through screens with microscopic pores. These devices work well, are reasonably affordable, and are particularly important if you live in a big city where fresh air is harder to come by.

Better yet, get an ionizer such as the Ionic Breeze (available at the Sharper Image; www.sharperimage.com). Perhaps you've noticed the air outside feels especially clean and fresh after a storm; that's because the air is filled with negative ions. When we seal off our homes to the environment, the ion content inside

TheGoalDiggerTip

Bang your drum.

Here's an odd way to boost your immunity, but it's a scientifically substantiated strategy nonetheless. According to a study conducted at the Mind-Body Wellness Center, an outpatient medical facility in Meadville, Pennsylvania, participating in group drumming sessions can result in increased activity of natural killer (NK) cells (the white blood cells that make up a major part of the immune system). "Drum circles have been part of healing rituals in many cultures throughout the world since antiquity," noted the researchers. "Drumming is a complex composite intervention with the potential to modulate specific neuroendocrine and neuroimmune parameters in a direction opposite to that expected with the classic stress response." In other words, grab a few buddies and break out the bongos, and you too can feel the therapeutic properties of percussion (and perhaps minimize anxiety). Much to the dismay of my wife, I drum regularly with my daughter, Vivienne—pots, pans, whatever—and this form of therapy works wonders for me and Viv. (Not sure about Brandy!)

can become unhealthful. A fair amount of research has shown that both the type and the quantity of ions in our air can have profound effects on our health. An ionizer can help reestablish a healthy balance of ions in your home.

Another way to cleanse the air indoors: Pick up some plants. "Houseplants, especially spider plants and Boston ferns, can help reduce formaldehyde and other airborne pollutants in your home," says Dr. Weil, who is a clinical professor of internal medicine and founder and director of the Program in Integrative Medicine at the University of Arizona in Tucson. As you may know, plants use carbon dioxide (CO_2) as fuel and release oxygen—the opposite of human metabolism (we breathe in oxygen and release CO_2). That's why plants don't just beautify your home but actually boost your health.

Be Social

In Chapter 5, I talked about how important spending time with others and having a support system can be for your confidence. But get this: Research shows that camaraderie and social interaction can have a positive impact on your immunity and that loneliness can impair it.

In one Ohio State University study, 227 women undergoing breast cancer treatment were divided into two groups—one that attended educational/support sessions and another that did not. At the end of 4 months, blood tests revealed that the women who had participated in the support sessions had higher levels of T cells (which help the body fight disease), while the women who did not attend the sessions showed no change in their T cell levels. In another study conducted at Carnegie Mellon University in Pittsburgh, first-year students who reported feelings of social isolation exhibited a weaker immune response to a first-time flu shot than students with a greater sense of social support. So much for independent spirit! It seems that John Donne was right when he said, "No man is an island ... "

Within this chapter, you've discovered many of the keys to unlocking a more injury- and illness-resistant body, primed and ready to perform with greater vitality and less pain. Now there's just one more thing your goal digger program cannot go without—and it's a biggie. Turn the page to learn how the foods you eat and the way you eat them won't just contribute to your fitness goals—be it weight management, improved performance, better health, greater energy, or all of the above—but truly send them soaring.

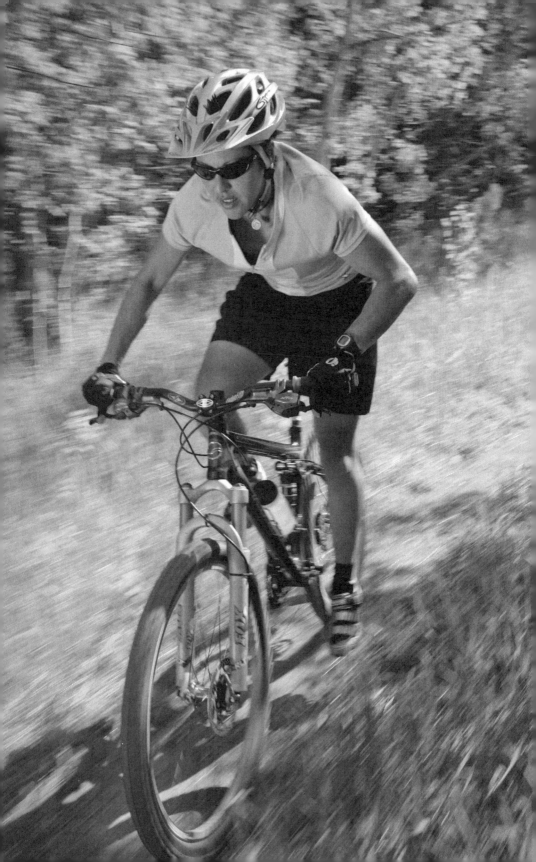

SEVEN

The Goal Digger Diet: Achieving Your Best via Optimum Eating

"Let your food be your medicine,
and your medicine be your food."
—Hippocrates

While the right types and amounts of exercise will help you achieve great things in your quest to recapture the athlete within, I'm sure you know that the right types and amounts of food are every bit as important. That said, a lot of people—goal diggers included—tend to focus exclusively, or at least disproportionately, on one aspect of their fitness (the diet *or* the exercise) rather than both, which, unfortunately, means they don't get the results they're after.

Of course, it can be tough to figure out what you're supposed to eat, how much of it, and when—particularly with all the fad diets perpetually flooding the market and all the "groundbreaking" research claiming to have

< 155 >

found a scientifically sound . . . new approach to eating or, better yet, a nutritional supplement that will give you . . . energy! . . . Weight loss! . . . Abs of Steel! . . . Buns of Topaz! . . . And all for just $49.99! . . . Try my product! From low carb to no carb to calorie restrictive to cabbage soup to detox diets, from metabolism-boosting to fat-burning miracle pills—it's easy to understand why you'd be a little confused about which methods (if any) will work best for you. I'd almost venture to say that, with the possible exception of superstring theory, nothing puzzles the intellect quite so much as the human diet. But it doesn't have to be this way.

In this chapter, I'm going to help you make sense of all the dietary minutiae. You'll probably be happy to hear that eating healthfully doesn't have to be complicated. In fact, *any* fitness goal you have will require the same basic principles, including an appropriate amount of calories to support your physiology and level of activity and the right balance of macronutrients (carbohydrates, proteins, and fats). From there, it's just a matter of making the best food choices within each category and timing things wisely throughout the day. Let's begin with some food fundamentals, then we'll get into more detail regarding how to make goal-specific tweaks and put it all together into the right meal plan for you.

OH CALORIES, MY CALORIES

You count them, you ration them, you may even do whatever you possibly can to burn them off—from cranking up your cardio workouts to eating more celery. Yes, whether you're trying to lose weight or simply maintain an optimum fitness level, chances are you view the poor little calorie with fear and loathing or, at the very least, confusion. But if you understand exactly what calories are and what they do, you can work with them rather than against them.

Simple truth: The calorie is not inherently evil. In nutritional terms, it is defined as a unit of energy-producing potential contained in food and released upon oxidation by the body. If we viewed calories this way—as fuel for our bodies, not unlike the insanely expensive gasoline we put into our cars—we might dramatically alter our relationship to the foods we eat and strive for the premium stuff that will keep us running smoothly and efficiently, rather than the cheap stuff that always seems to require we go in for an extra tune-up when we haven't driven nearly enough miles.

Okay, enough with the car analogies. My point is that you should be

The**GoalDigger**Tip

Find a food coach.

In the first chapter, I talked about the importance of enlisting a professional—a personal trainer—to help you reach your workout goals, particularly if you're not entirely sure what you should be doing. If your head is spinning from all the eat-right information I'm providing in this chapter—or if you're simply dumbfounded by all things relating to diet (and these days, who isn't?!)—you should also seek out a registered dietetic professional. To find someone with the appropriate educational background and credentials, visit the American Dietetic Association's Web site at www.eatright.org, and click on "Find a Nutrition Professional."

intent upon fueling your body as effectively as possible, and to do that, you must get to know the caloric breakdown of the foods you consume, and aim for the appropriate quantities.

Let's look at the big picture first: How many calories should you consume each day? That depends on your height, weight, age, gender, body composition (how much fat and muscle you have), general health, genetics, and how much exercise you get. Believe it or not, there is a formula known as the Harris-Benedict equation that takes a lot of these factors into account and can therefore give you a fairly good estimate of your basal metabolic rate (BMR)—which is how many calories your body burns at rest (or the minimum number you need to maintain your basic bodily processes, not counting exercise, each day). Using that number, another formula considers your activity levels, which will help determine approximately how many calories you'll need each day while doing the 14-Day Programs. First, here's the formula for your BMR.

FOR MEN, YOUR BMR =

66 + (6.23 × your weight in pounds) + (12.7 × your height in inches) − (6.8 × your age in years)

FOR WOMEN, YOUR BMR =

655 + (4.35 × your weight in pounds) + (4.7 × your height in inches) − (4.7 × your age in years)

To give you an example: Let's say you're a 25-year-old male, 180 pounds and 6 feet tall (or 72 inches). That's 66 + (6.23 × 180) + (12.7 × 72) − (6.8 × 25) = 66 + 1,121 + 914 − 170 = 1,931.

So, your BMR—the number of calories your body requires just to sit around doing next to nothing—is 1,931.

Now that you know your BMR, you can multiply that by one of the following numbers to determine how many additional calories you'll need to consume to maintain the activity you'll be getting.

If you're sedentary (little or no exercise): Multiply by 1.2.

If you're lightly active (light exercise/sports 1 to 3 days/week): Multiply by 1.375.

If you're moderately active (moderate exercise/sports 3 to 5 days/week): multiply by 1.55.

If you're very active (hard exercise/sports 6 or 7 days a week): Multiply by 1.725.

If you're extra active (very hard exercise/sports and physical job): Multiply by 1.9.

Given these figures, here's what you should do for the 14-Day Programs.

If you're doing the Energize and/or Time-Saver workouts, multiply your BMR by 1.55.

If you're doing the Challenge and/or Full-Fledged workouts, multiply your BMR by 1.725.

If you're doing the advanced, Challenge, *and* Full-Fledged workouts, multiply your BMR by 1.9.

For example, the previous 25-year-old male doing the intermediate Challenge Program should be consuming 3,331 calories a day (1,931 × 1.725); that's 1,400 extra calories a day!

I know this seems like a lot of math—but I wanted you to have the formulas in case you're a numbers junkie. If you're not, you can *still* figure out your daily caloric needs by visiting any number of Web sites with BMR and caloric needs calculators. For example, check out www.bcm.edu/cnrc/

caloriesneed.htm and punch in the "about 1 hour/day" answer to the question "Are you active?" If you punch in the numbers I gave you for the 25-year-old man, you'll see that the resulting calorie needs figure is pretty close—within 50 calories—to the one we calculated above.

You may be wondering why that number is so important. While I don't want you to fixate on calories, I do want you to get a sense of how many are required to fuel the amount of exercise you'll be getting while pushing your fitness to greater heights on the 14-Day Programs. Clearly, you're going to be putting in a lot of hard work, and the last thing you want to do is deprive yourself of the calories you need to fuel that work.

Why? Several reasons. First, if you deprive yourself of too many calories, your metabolic rate slows, which is an act of self-preservation. Your body is essentially saying, "You're not feeding me enough, and in case we're starving here, I'm going into conservation mode." Then, of course, when you eat as much as you actually need, your body responds by storing every available spare calorie as body fat—just in case you decide to "semistarve" yourself again.

Beyond that, if you restrict your calories, your performance suffers, you risk injuries, and, instead of maintaining muscle mass and losing body fat, you lose both, says Cynthia Sass, RD, a registered dietitian in Tampa, a spokesperson for the American Dietetic Association, and coauthor of *Your Diet Is Driving Me Crazy: When Food Conflicts Get in the Way of Your Love Life*. In a nutshell: You won't accomplish any goal, whether it's looking, feeling, or performing better or improving your health, if you don't get enough fuel.

It should also go without saying that if you consume too many calories, your body stores them as fat—so it's important to take in only as many calories as your body needs. One pound of fat equals 3,500 calories. That may sound like a lot, but if you have just 100 extra calories a day (found in about 1 tablespoon of butter, an egg, a slice of bread, or one banana, for example), you'll gain a pound every 5 weeks—or just over 10 pounds in a year!

If your goal is to lose weight, experts recommend that you do so at a slow rate: Specifically, aim to drop no more than a pound or two a week. Since, as I just explained, a pound of fat equals 3,500 calories, you simply need to aim for 500 to 1,000 fewer calories each day than the calorie needs you determined for yourself above. If, for example, our 25-year-old man eats between 2,331 and 2,881 calories a day—rather than the 3,331 required to maintain his weight—he'll lose 1 to 2 pounds a week. He'll still get quite a lot of calories, and since he's getting plenty of exercise, there's little danger of the body going into conservation mode.

Getting pretty close to your target number of calories each day is important—but of course there's more to fueling your body than that. Those calories need to be an appropriate balance of macronutrients—and that's what we'll address next.

CARBOS AND PROTEINS AND FATS—OH MY!

Sure, the Atkins-crazed, high-protein proponents who become hysterical if forced to so much as look at a loaf of bread have once again faded into the fad-diet woodwork, but there are still a lot of misconceptions about the

Vitamins for Vitality

I'm sure you know that vitamins and minerals are crucial for health, performance, and looking and feeling your best. Ideally, you get the bulk of your vitamins and minerals from the foods you eat; to do so, focus on getting a balance of macronutrients from the food sources recommended in this chapter. However, you may still end up short, so it wouldn't hurt to take a daily multivitamin. Research suggests that these supplements may help prevent chronic disease and even help your athletic performance if taken regularly (not if you only pop one just before a workout!).

A multivitamin can also protect you from becoming deficient in any one nutrient, which can lead to low energy levels; that's because vitamins and minerals are involved in many of the chemical reactions that release energy from fuels. Some of the B vitamins, for example, act as shuttle buses to move carbohydrates through the process of breakdown into energy. If you're short on any one of the Bs, the process can slow down. You can get all the Bs you need in a good multi. As a guide, look for one that has about 30 milligrams of B_6, 400 to 800 micrograms of folic acid, and 100 micrograms of B_{12}. It should also contain at least 200 milligrams of magnesium.

The minerals magnesium and iron also play major roles in energy production. Iron, for example, transports oxygen throughout the body. People who are short on either mineral are tired and lack endurance. Even though iron is important, however, experts recommend supplemental iron

three macronutrients, how much of each you should ideally consume each day, and why. I'll give you the bottom line right out of the gate: You need to get 45 to 65 percent of your daily calories from carbohydrates, 20 to 35 percent from fat, and 10 to 35 percent from protein. This is according to the National Academies of Sciences' Institute of Medicine, as well as just about any dietitian or nutritionist worth the paper his or her certification is printed on.

Why should you be shooting for these ranges? First, they collectively provide virtually all your caloric energy (specifically, 1 gram of carbohydrates has 4 calories, 1 gram of protein has 4 calories, and 1 gram of fat has 9 calories), and you use all three, in varying degrees, to fuel your basic physiological functions as well as your exercise. Your metabolism is cranking

only to certain groups of people—primarily premenopausal women, who lose iron every month during menstruation and have a hard time making it up. If you're in that group, don't take more than 18 milligrams of supplemental iron a day without a doctor's diagnosis of your iron status. If a blood test shows that you have low iron levels, your doctor will prescribe a supplement, perhaps in a large dose, to get you back on course. You'll be pleasantly surprised at how much more energy you'll soon have!

Athletes can also lose a bit of iron through sweat or the breakdown of blood cells caused by impact from activities like running. Muscles also have a high demand for iron-containing molecules in their cells. Still, most men don't require supplemental iron and shouldn't take it; too much iron can be harmful.

Vitamin E deserves special mention because it helps to reduce the damage to muscles that can cause delayed soreness after intense exercise—a problem almost every athlete over age 50 knows about. It's called oxidative damage. One study showed that taking 300 milligrams of vitamin E daily reduced exercise-induced oxidative damage in cyclists. I suggest you get this amount in your multi or take a separate supplement, preferably one that contains natural mixed tocopherols, including tocotrienol (scientific names for forms of vitamin E). Nuts, seeds, and wheat germ are also good food sources of vitamin E.

along—and you're burning calories—even when you're at rest. During those times, your body gets slightly more than half of its energy from fats and most of the rest from carbohydrates, along with a small percentage from proteins. When you're exercising, the mixture of fuels is modified—and the amounts of each one used depend on how long and how hard you're working out as well as the sort of shape you're in (how well you're conditioned to be doing the activity you're doing).

But there's more to it than energy supply. While carbohydrates are your most efficient source of energy, protein is not only used for energy but broken down into amino acids and reassembled into whatever proteins your body needs to make muscle, bone, skin, hair, and all the connective tissues that literally keep you from falling apart. Certain amino acids found in protein are considered essential, meaning your body can't make them; you can only get them from food. And then there's fat, which isn't all bad, no matter how awful the word may sound to you. In addition to providing you with energy, fats help your body to make cell membranes and certain hormones and to absorb the fat-soluble vitamins A, E, D, and K. Like amino acids, some fats are considered essential and can be obtained only from specific food sources.

Clearly, all three macronutrients are important components of a healthy diet. You need a good balance of carbs, proteins, and fats each and every day, but what are the best sources of each? We'll take a look at that now.

Let's Talk about Carbs, Baby

You've probably heard a lot about "good carbs" and "bad carbs" lately—as well as "complex" and "simple" ones. But none of these labels are likely helping you figure out if that bowl of oatmeal you had for breakfast was your best bet or if you should be bolting toward or away from the bagel shop.

There are two primary forms of carbohydrates: simple sugars (aka simple carbohydrates), which are found in things like fruit (fructose), milk (lactose), and table sugar (sucrose); and starches (aka complex carbohydrates), found in foods like rice, potatoes, legumes, breads, and cereals. No matter what kind of carbohydrates you consume, they'll be converted to a simple sugar called glucose, which is then either stored in the muscles or absorbed into the bloodstream. As your blood sugar rises, your pancreas releases a hormone called insulin—necessary for moving glucose from the blood into the cells, where it can be used for energy.

So if all carbs are converted into simple sugar, why are some considered good and others bad? There are a couple factors: how quickly the foods you eat cause your blood sugar levels to rise and how nutrient-rich the foods are. Generally, you should avoid simple sugars and refined or processed foods—things like sugary sodas, candy, doughnuts, products made with white flour, white rice, and pasta—because they don't contain fiber and other essential nutrients; they're basically empty calories. Beyond that, because they're so simple and the body doesn't need to break them down, they enter the bloodstream quickly—and if you eat too many at once, they tend to cause a rapid rise in blood sugar, which research indicates may increase your risk for health issues like diabetes and heart disease, as well as obesity. The quick energy spike is also often followed by an equally quick decline, which can cause fatigue and hunger and generally makes you feel miserable.

The**GoalDigger**Tip

Fill up on fiber.

The American Dietetic Association (ADA) recommends that healthy adults get 20 to 35 grams of dietary fiber a day, depending on caloric intake (e.g., if you're consuming 2,000 calories a day, you should consume 25 grams of fiber)—but research suggests the average American only consumes 14 to 15 grams.

What's so fabulous about fiber and why should you be ramping up the roughage? "Long heralded as part of a healthy diet, fiber appears to reduce the risk of developing various conditions, including heart disease, diabetes, diverticular disease, and constipation," says the Harvard School of Public Health. The two principal types of dietary fiber are soluble and insoluble. The former is believed to help reduce blood cholesterol levels, while the latter aids in digestion and removing waste and toxins from your body—keeping your gastrointestinal tract healthy. Good sources of soluble fiber include legumes, potatoes, and oats, while sources of insoluble fiber include bran, nuts, and seeds; both types are found in a lot of fruits and vegetables.

Your best bet is to opt for nutritious sources of simple carbs, like fruit (which usually provides fiber) and low-fat or nonfat dairy products, as well as nutrient and fiber-rich complex carbs, like whole grain breads, cereals and pastas, brown rice, legumes (foods found in pods, like beans and peas), and vegetables. These foods will help you achieve all your goals: Since they're broken down more slowly, they help you feel full so you won't overeat, and they provide a steadier stream of energy so you feel and perform better; plus, they're your best choices for overall health (particularly fiber; see "Fill Up on Fiber" on page 163).

MyPyramid, the food guide promoted by the American Dietetic Association (ADA), recommends a range of servings in each food group that, if followed, will help you easily get your target percentage of carbs each day. Those guidelines are as follows:

- Bread, cereal, rice, and pasta: 6 to 11 servings
- Vegetables: 3 to 5 servings
- Fruits: 2 to 4 servings
- Milk, yogurt, and cheese: 2 to 3 servings
- Meat, poultry, fish, dry beans, eggs, and nuts: 2 to 3 servings
- Fats, oils, and sweets: Use sparingly.

Should You Carbo-Load for Better Performance?

Because some athletes work at high intensities or extended durations (more than an hour), they will sometimes do what's known as carbo-loading—getting about 70 percent of their daily calories from carbohydrates. While this may indeed trick your muscles into storing extra glycogen (strings of glucose) before a competition, it's not necessary for the average athlete—even if you're on a quest to boost your workout performance. Simply getting about 50 percent of your calories from carbohydrates should fuel your fitness perfectly. You can certainly play with the numbers—going as high as 65 percent carbs—and see if it impacts your ability to perform, but you absolutely don't need to go any higher than that. It's all about experimenting to figure out what works for you, while still maintaining the balance experts recommend.

For more information on MyPyramid and what constitutes a serving, visit the ADA Web site at www.eatright.org.

Protein Power!

Like carbs, protein has won and lost favor many times over in the fad diet world. But, as mentioned earlier, it is an essential macronutrient, partly for the fuel it provides and largely because of its structural and functional roles. When you eat protein, the body breaks it down and converts it into amino acids and peptides (chains of amino acids), which are then absorbed into the bloodstream. The body requires about 20 amino acids for normal functioning, and nine of them are considered essential (your body cannot make them and must get them from the foods you eat).

So what are the best ways to get those essential amino acids? Animal sources—meat, eggs, and dairy products—generally provide a better balance than vegetable sources. (Eggs are as close to a perfect protein as you can get.) That doesn't mean you can't survive on vegetable proteins; it just means you need to mix and match vegetable sources to get a good balance—the old rice-and-beans routine.

If you're a vegetarian, you may need to supplement your diet with a protein powder drink as a snack or even a meal. Protein powders can be beneficial because they allow you to add protein to your diet without adding a lot of fat or extra calories. Soy protein offers lots of health benefits, including lowering your risk for heart disease and certain cancers. It can also help lower cholesterol. However, some people say rice protein powders are easier to digest than soy- or whey-based powders. Try all three and see which works best for you.

You've probably also heard that you need extra protein to build muscle and fuel your strength-training exercise. This is true, to a degree. If you're doing a high-intensity resistance-training workout designed to build muscle (which may be true of some of the sport-specific training you do in the Perform Better Program, for instance), you could add up to an ounce of body protein to existing muscle mass each day. For this reason, you'll need to eat a little more protein—but no more than the maximum of 35 percent of calories that experts recommend.

Here's an easy way to calculate how much protein you should be consuming: Divide your weight in pounds by 2.2 to get your weight in kilograms.

Then multiply that by 1 and 1.5 to find your daily protein range in grams. If you weigh 160 pounds, for example, your daily protein range is 73 to 109 grams—the equivalent of about 10 to 15 ounces of meat (since an ounce of meat contains about 7 grams of protein). When picking your protein sources, make sure you're opting for the leanest and lowest-fat versions possible.

Fat Is Not a Four-Letter Word

Of all the macronutrients, fat has perhaps come under the greatest fire—and as with carbohydrates, there are fats that are considered "bad" and others that are "good." Let's talk first about the fats you should limit in your diet: saturated and trans fats. Research shows that consuming these types of fats raises LDL (bad) cholesterol and lowers HDL (good) cholesterol, and that in turn increases your risk for coronary heart disease—one of the leading causes of death in the United States.

Saturated fats are found in meats—especially cuts that have solid, visible pieces of white fat and/or skin (like poultry)—as well as in butter, lard, coconut and palm oil, and high-fat dairy products like whole milk, cream, and cheese. Trans fats are hydrogenated oils that preserve the shelf life and flavor of foods; they're in vegetable shortenings, certain margarines, cookies, crackers, and other snack foods. Doughnuts, pastries, and a lot of fried foods are also high in trans fats, and there are small amounts in some meats and dairy products. The FDA, which estimates that the average American over age 20 consumes about 5.8 grams of trans fats (or 2.6 percent of calories) each day, recently required that trans fats be listed on food labels; saturated fat has been required since 1993. So read those labels, and limit your intake accordingly!

On a happier note, we do require some fat, and we can only get certain types our body needs—like linoleic and linolenic—from the foods we eat. These "good" fats are known as monounsaturated and polyunsaturated and are generally found in plant oils like safflower, sesame, sunflower, corn, and soybean; in olive, peanut, and canola oils; and in avocados. Fatty fish like salmon is also a good source (specifically, it provides "omega-3" polyunsaturated fat—all the rage among the health-conscious set these days). Unlike saturated fats that may cause heart disease, studies show that these kinds may actually *prevent* it—along with lowering your risk for developing cardiovascular disease and certain types of cancer. In fact, polyunsaturated fat is the best fat for you and should be a part of every healthy diet.

TIMING YOUR FOOD INTAKE

Now you know what you should be eating and how much—but *when* you eat is also important, particularly for maintaining your energy levels and fueling your exercise. It can also impact things like weight management; if you tend to skip a meal, you may wind up overeating (and even eating less healthfully) when you finally do make your way to the fridge or, worse yet, the fast-food drive-thru.

Your best bet is to make sure you don't let too many hours go by without eating. "Don't go any more than 5 hours between meals or snacks," advises Sass. "This can cause fatigue, low blood sugar, and loss of lean tissue." It can also send your metabolism into conservation mode, as I mentioned earlier. As far as fueling your workouts, I've found that it's best to have a snack 1 to 2 hours before exercise. This allows you to start with enough glucose in your bloodstream to get you going and keep you going without feeling weak or shaky.

Your preworkout snack should be 200 to 300 calories (up to 400 calories, depending on your daily calorie intake) and provide mostly carbohydrates, along with some protein or fat. See the One-Day Meal Plans beginning on page 170 for goal-specific preworkout snack suggestions.

You should also make it a point to drink water before you exercise, especially if you sweat a lot. You'd be surprised how much even a little dehydration can contribute to a fatigue; it actually makes it harder for your blood to deliver oxygen to your muscles and can make your arms and legs feel heavy. In general, you should drink before you feel thirsty; believe it or not, you can lose up to 2 percent of your body weight as sweat or urine before your thirst mechanism even sets in! If you tend to sweat a lot, you may need 10 to 12 glasses (8 ounces each) of fluid a day. Here's a simple four-step fluid schedule to help you stay properly hydrated.

- Two hours before you exercise, drink 3 cups (24 ounces) of fluid.

- Ten to 15 minutes before you exercise, drink 2 cups (16 ounces).

- Every 15 minutes during exercise, drink 1 cup (8 ounces).

- After exercise, drink 2 cups (16 ounces).

You can also weigh yourself before and after a workout to see how much fluid you've lost and thus need to replenish. One pound of body weight equals roughly 2 cups (16 ounces) of fluid.

The**GoalDigger**Tip

Slow down, you eat too fast.

While the sample meal plans in this chapter—and the ones found at www.whfoods.com—will provide you with excellent, fast, and easy ways to fuel your fitness goals, there's an important lesson taught at health resorts and spas around the world, and it's one we could all benefit from: Put more time and energy into the foods you eat.

"We are trying to get people to redefine their relationship to food—from organic gardening to eating more local, seasonal organics to eating a broader variety of foods to conscious cooking to mindful eating," explains Yvonne Nienstadt, nutrition director for Rancho La Puerta Fitness Resort & Spa in Tecate, Baja California, Mexico. "We want people to find joy in the kitchen and to eat the food they have prepared in a calm and slow manner to enhance digestion and assimilation. Alas, for the most part, our culture does not support this ideal."

You don't have to get all those fluids from water; sports drinks such as Gatorade contain half the sugar of sweetened teas, sodas, or fruit drinks, along with small amounts of sodium and potassium, two minerals lost during sweating—so they are a decent choice. Even so, the calories start to add up if you have too many sports drinks, so stick to no more than 16 ounces a day, even on heavy training days, and get most of your fluids from water.

It's also important to have a good recovery meal or snack as soon as possible after intense exercise. Sass notes that she often sees athletes who don't want to eat after training lest they "put back what they just burned"—but that's a bad idea. "You'll only put back body fat if you eat a recovery meal with too many calories," she says. "But not enough calories can increase the risk of injury or negatively impact performance. You need carbohydrate to replenish glycogen, protein to repair muscle and bone, some healthy fat (also for repair), fluid to replace sweat loss, and vitamins and minerals to replenish what was used during exercise and to aid in healing." See the One-Day Meal Plans starting on page 170 for goal-specific postworkout snack suggestions.

That's why, in addition to the meal plans outlined in this chapter, I've compiled recipes from some of North America's greatest destinations—Rancho La Puerta, as well as Red Mountain Spa in St. George, Utah, and Lake Austin Spa Resort in Austin, Texas. These phenomenal places cater to people who are working to take their fitness to the next level. Guests ramp up their activity levels, work on maximizing their energy and performance, and strive for greater overall health. Master chefs on staff cook all the meals, but the hope is that people will take the nutritional lessons they've learned during their stay and incorporate them into their own lives. Turn to page 197 to explore the delicious recipes the chefs from these spas have so kindly contributed to this book, and start including them in your diet today!

MAKE A MEAL OF IT

Now that we've addressed all the details regarding calories, macronutrients, and ideal foods for fueling your active lifestyle, it's time to put this information into practice. To that end, the following One-Day Meal Plans were created by Melina B. Jampolis, MD, a board-certified internist and one of only 198 physician nutrition specialists in the U.S. (who is also host of the Discovery Network's FIT TV series *Diet Doctor*). If your goal is to look or feel better, try the menu that targets both of those objectives. Likewise, follow the meal plan for either improved performance if that's your primary goal, or for improved health if that's your number one target. (Of course, because these are all great meal plans that will benefit your body in a variety of ways, there's no reason you can't try them all!) Within each goal are three different caloric targets to help you meet your daily needs—so select your plan accordingly. If you find you need even more calories than prescribed here, add two additional servings of vegetables and up to two extra servings of lean, quality proteins. Remember to listen to your body above all else.

You should also note that these are simply leaping-off points that should be used as examples; give them a try, then explore a variety of healthy options and incorporate them into your own personalized menus as you learn which foods you like best and which ones help you achieve your personal best. For additional ideas—including quick and delicious recipes and weekly meal plans designed to help you prevent or manage specific illnesses and diseases, manage your weight, and boost your energy to boot—I highly recommend a fantastic Web site called the World's Healthiest Foods: www. whfoods.com.

THE ONE-DAY MEAL PLANS: WEIGHT LOSS AND INCREASED ENERGY

This menu includes protein with every meal and snack to help rev your metabolism, fill you up, and preserve lean body mass as you lose weight, notes Jampolis. Meanwhile, the high-fiber, low glycemic index carbohydrates (fruits, vegetables, beans, brown rice, high-fiber bread) keep your blood sugar stable and give you a steady release of energy throughout the day. The fiber also helps keep you fuller, making it easier to cut calories slightly (these daily targets are 200 calories lower than the other goal-specific plans) for weight loss.

CALORIC GOAL: 1,600
(45% CARBS, 30% PROTEIN, 25% FAT)

Breakfast

1 whole egg plus 2 egg whites, scrambled (110 calories)

1 slice high-fiber toast (3 grams fiber minimum) (90 calories)

1 tablespoon peanut butter (90 calories)

½ cup fruit (60 calories)

1 cup coffee with ¼ cup skim milk (20 calories)

Total calories: 370

Lunch

Healthy chicken taco salad:

2 cups romaine lettuce (25 calories)

3 ounces skinless chicken (105 calories)

½ cup black beans (120 calories)

¼ cup low-fat shredded cheese (60 calories)

½ cup salsa (as dressing) (45 calories)

Total calories: 355

Dinner

5 ounces of white fish (150 calories)

2 cups veggies (50 calories)

1 tablespoon olive oil (100 calories)

½ cup brown rice (90 calories)

Healthy Choice Fudgsicle (90 calories)

Total calories: 480

Pre-Workout Snack

⅛ cup almonds (85 calories)

1 medium apple (80 calories)

Total calories: 165

Post-Workout Snack

Protein Bar (10–14 grams protein, at least 3 grams fiber) (200 calories)

Total calories: 200

TOTAL CALORIES FOR DAY: 1,580

CALORIC GOAL: 1,800
(45% CARBS, 30% PROTEIN, 25% FAT)

Breakfast

1 whole egg plus 2 egg whites, scrambled (110 calories)

1 slice high-fiber toast (3 grams fiber minimum) (90 calories)

1 tablespoon peanut butter (90 calories)

½ cup fruit (60 calories)

1 cup coffee with ¼ cup skim milk (20 calories)

Total calories: 370

Lunch

Healthy chicken taco salad:

2 cups romaine lettuce (25 calories)

4 ounces skinless chicken (150 calories)

½ cup black beans (120 calories)

¼ cup low-fat shredded cheese (60 calories)

½ cup salsa (as dressing) (45 calories)

Total calories: 400

Dinner

5 ounces of white fish (150 calories)

2 cups veggies (50 calories)

1 tablespoon olive oil (100 calories)

1 cup brown rice (180 calories)

Healthy Choice Fudgsicle (90 calories)

Total calories: 570

Pre-Workout Snack

¼ cup almonds (170 calories)

1 medium apple (80 calories)

Total calories: 150

Post-Workout Snack

Protein Bar (10–14 grams protein, at least 3 grams fiber) (200 calories)

Total calories: 200

TOTAL CALORIES FOR DAY: 1,790

CALORIC GOAL: 2,000
(45% CARBS, 30% PROTEIN, 25% FAT)

Breakfast

1 whole egg plus 2 egg whites, scrambled (110 calories)

2 slices high-fiber toast (3 grams fiber minimum per slice) (180 calories)

1 tablespoon peanut butter (90 calories)

½ cup fruit (60 calories)

1 cup coffee with ¼ cup skim milk (20 calories)

Total calories: 450

Lunch

Healthy chicken taco salad:

2 cups romaine lettuce (25 calories)

5 ounces skinless chicken (185 calories)

¾ cup black beans (180 calories)

¼ cup low-fat shredded cheese (60 calories)

½ cup salsa (as dressing) (45 calories)

Total calories: 495

Dinner

6 ounces of white fish (180 calories)

2 cups veggies (50 calories)

1 tablespoon olive oil (100 calories)

1 cup brown rice (180 calories)

Healthy Choice Fudgsicle (90 calories)

Total calories: 600

Pre-Workout Snack

¼ cup almonds (170 calories)

1 medium apple (80 calories)

Total calories: 250

Post-Workout Snack

Protein Bar (10–14 grams protein, at least 3 grams fiber) (200 calories)

Total calories: 200

TOTAL CALORIES FOR DAY: 1,995

THE ONE-DAY MEAL PLANS: PERFORM BETTER

This menu emphasizes a slightly higher percentage of carbohydrates throughout the day—and particularly prior to your workout—to fuel your activity levels, says Jampolis. The pre-workout banana is a higher glycemic index carbohydrate that gives the body faster acting fuel for your performance. The protein smoothie post-workout helps replenish muscle glycogen and protect your muscle, Jampolis notes. Large amounts of fruits, vegetables, and good fats (avocado, peanut) also help ensure your cells are developing in a nutrient-rich environment, she adds.

CALORIC GOAL: 1,800
(55% CARBS, 20% PROTEIN, 25% FAT)

Breakfast

1 cup cooked oatmeal with 2 teaspoons brown sugar (175 calories)

½ cup blueberries (60 calories)

½ cup low-fat cottage cheese (120 calories)

Coffee with ½ cup skim milk (45 calories)

Total calories: 400

Lunch

Turkey avocado sandwich:

3 ounces turkey (120 calories)

¼ avocado (50 calories)

2 slices whole grain bread (180 calories)

1 ounce pretzels (100 calories)

Total calories: 450

Dinner

4-ounce skinless chicken breast (160 calories)

1 medium-sized baked sweet potato (120 calories)

1 cup cooked broccoli sprinkled with 1 tablespoon fresh grated parmesan (100 calories)

1 cup plain yogurt with cinnamon and Splenda (110 calories)

Total calories: 490

Pre-Workout Snack

Large banana (120 calories)

1½ tablespoons peanut butter (120 calories)

Total calories: 240

Post-Workout Snack

Smoothie:

1 cup skim milk (100 calories)

1 scoop whey protein (90 calories)

½ cup frozen fruit (30 calories)

Total calories: 220

TOTAL CALORIES FOR DAY: 1,800

CALORIC GOAL: 2,000
(55% CARBS, 20% PROTEIN, 25% FAT)

Breakfast

1½ cups cooked oatmeal with 2 teaspoons brown sugar (250 calories)

½ cup blueberries (60 calories)

½ cup low-fat cottage cheese (120 calories)

Coffee with ½ cup skim milk (45 calories)

Total calories: 475

Lunch

Turkey avocado sandwich:

3 ounces turkey (120 calories)

½ avocado (100 calories)

2 slices whole grain bread (180 calories)

1 ounce pretzels (100 calories)

Total calories: 500

Dinner

5-ounce skinless chicken breast (200 calories)

1 medium-sized baked sweet potato (120 calories)

1 cup cooked broccoli sprinkled with 1 tablespoon fresh grated parmesan (100 calories)

1 cup plain yogurt with cinnamon and Splenda (110 calories)

Total calories: 530

Pre-Workout Snack

Large banana (120 calories)

1½ tablespoons peanut butter (120 calories)

Total calories: 240

Post-Workout Snack

Smoothie:

1 cup skim milk (100 calories)

1 scoop whey protein (90 calories)

1 cup frozen fruit (60 calories)

Total calories: 250

TOTAL CALORIES FOR DAY: 1,995

CALORIC GOAL: 2,200
(55% CARBS, 20% PROTEIN, 25% FAT)

Breakfast

1½ cups cooked oatmeal with 2 teaspoons brown sugar (250 calories)

½ cup blueberries (60 calories)

½ cup low-fat cottage cheese (120 calories)

Coffee with ½ cup skim milk (45 calories)

Total calories: 475

Lunch

Turkey avocado sandwich:

4 ounces turkey (160 calories)

½ avocado (100 calories)

2 slices whole grain bread (180 calories)

1 ounce pretzels (100 calories)

Total calories: 540

Dinner

6-ounce skinless chicken breast (240 calories)

1 medium-sized baked sweet potato (120 calories)

1 cup cooked broccoli sprinkled with 1 tablespoon fresh grated parmesan (100 calories)

1 whole wheat dinner roll (120 calories)

1 cup plain yogurt with cinnamon and Splenda (110 calories)

Total calories: 690

Pre-Workout Snack

Large banana (120 calories)

1½ tablespoons peanut butter (120 calories)

Total calories: 240

Post-Workout Snack

Smoothie:

1 cup skim milk (100 calories)

1 scoop whey protein (90 calories)

1 cup frozen fruit (60 calories)

Total calories: 250

TOTAL CALORIES FOR DAY: 2,195

THE ONE-DAY MEAL PLANS: BETTER HEALTH

These meals are based on "The Alternative Healthy Eating Index," which prescribes five servings of vegetables, four servings of fruit, one serving of nuts or soy, a 4:1 ratio of white-to-red meat, 15 grams of cereal fiber, and high levels of unsaturated fats (nuts, olive oil) compared to saturated fats, along with a moderate amount of alcohol (1 serving for women, 2 for men). This way of eating has been associated with markedly lower levels of inflammation in the body—potentially decreasing your risks for cancer, heart disease, and diabetes, along with a host of inflammation-related illnesses, says Jampolis.

CALORIC GOAL: 1,800
(50% CARBS, 20% PROTEIN, 30% FAT)

Breakfast

1½ cups Kashi GO LEAN cereal (135 calories)

1 cup skim milk (90 calories)

½ cup blueberries (60 calories)

2 tablespoons slivered almonds (90 calories)

1 cup green tea (0 calories)

Total calories: 375

Lunch

3-ounce skinless chicken breast (120 calories)

1 cup brown rice (180 calories)

1 cup spinach (25 calories)

2 teaspoons olive oil (50 calories)

1 small apple (60 calories)

Total calories: 435

Dinner

4 ounces salmon (225 calories)

1 cup lentils (180 calories)

1 cup cooked carrots (50 calories)

1 5-ounce glass red wine (120 calories)

½ cup fresh fruit (60 calories)

Total calories: 635

Pre-Workout Snack

1 cup plain yogurt (with cinnamon and Splenda, if desired)
(110 calories)

½ cup high-fiber, low-fat granola (90 calories)

Total calories: 200

Post-Workout Snack

⅛ cup almonds (85 calories)

1 orange (80 calories)

Total calories: 165

TOTAL CALORIES FOR DAY: 1,810

CALORIC GOAL: 2,000
(50% CARBS, 20% PROTEIN, 30% FAT)

Breakfast

1½ cups Kashi GO LEAN cereal (135 calories)

1 cup skim milk (90 calories)

½ cup blueberries (60 calories)

2 tablespoons slivered almonds (90 calories)

1 cup green tea (0 calories)

Total calories: 375

Lunch

4-ounce skinless chicken breast (160 calories)

1 cup brown rice (180 calories)

1 cup spinach (25 calories)

2 teaspoons olive oil (50 calories)

1 small apple (60 calories)

Total calories: 475

Dinner

5 ounces salmon (275 calories)

1 cup lentils (180 calories)

1 cup cooked carrots (50 calories)

1 5-ounce glass red wine (120 calories)

½ cup fresh fruit (60 calories)

Total calories: 685

Pre-Workout Snack

1 cup plain yogurt (with cinnamon and Splenda, optional) (110 calories)

½ cup high-fiber, low-fat granola (90 calories)

Total calories: 200

Post-Workout Snack

¼ cup almonds (170 calories)

1 orange (80 calories)

Total calories: 250

TOTAL CALORIES FOR DAY: 1,985

CALORIC GOAL: 2,200
(50% CARBS, 20% PROTEIN, 30% FAT)

Breakfast

2 cups Kashi GO LEAN cereal (180 calories)

1 cup skim milk (90 calories)

½ cup blueberries (60 calories)

2 tablespoons slivered almonds (90 calories)

1 cup green tea (0 calories)

Total calories: 420

Lunch

5-ounce skinless chicken breast (200 calories)

1 cup brown rice (180 calories)

1 cup spinach (25 calories)

2 teaspoons olive oil (50 calories)

1 small apple (60 calories)

Total calories: 515

Dinner

5 ounces salmon (275 calories)

1 cup lentils (180 calories)

1 cup cooked carrots (50 calories)

1 5-ounce glass red wine (120 calories)*

1 cup fresh fruit (120 calories)*

Total calories: 745

Pre-Workout Snack

1 cup plain yogurt (with cinnamon and Splenda, optional) (110 calories)

¾ cup high-fiber, low fat granola (135 calories)

Total calories: 245

Post-Workout Snack

¼ cup almonds (170 calories)

1 orange (80 calories)

Total calories: 250

TOTAL CALORIES FOR DAY: 2,175

Wine-lovers' option: Have ½ cup of fruit instead of one cup, and instead have a second 5-ounce glass of wine for a dinner calorie total of 805 and a daily calorie total of 2,225

Appendix 1
Goal Digger Logs

Regularly recording the reasons for the exercise you do will ensure you stay motivated—and the deeper and more powerful your reasons, the more consistent and inspired you'll be! As discussed in Chapter 2, you need to be as detailed as possible about what you want and how you're going to get it, while also homing in on what's realistic for you. Filling out these logs can help.

GOAL DIGGER LOG

The last time I was as active as I wanted to be was:

_____

_____

_____

< 183 >

What's motivating me now to take on greater fitness challenges:

I want to go out with
_Bianca Huff or ___ but_
get into shape for both of them!!!

The obstacles I may face in my quest for greater fitness include:

lazyness, lack of motivation,
_not sure ___ food ____
& sweats

The ways I can overcome these obstacles are as follows:

Get better sleep. Get a picture with
an image I want to match, don't
buy snacks or sodas.

The specific results I'd like to see—physically, mentally, emotionally, or otherwise—are as follows:

I want to lose weight & get a
six-pack & I want to feel good
every time I take my shirt off

When I accomplish all of these goals, I will be:

I will be really happy & I will
try getting Bianca or Negrota to
like me.

I know my goals are realistic because:

Because it's just a matter of
time & effort in order to
accomplish them.

GOAL DIGGER LOOK BETTER LOG:

The last time I was happy with my physique was:

_____

_____

_____

What's motivating me now to achieve my all-time best body:

_____

_____

_____

By the end of my first 14-Day Look Better Program, I want to see the following changes in my physique:

_____

_____

_____

After completing my first 14-Day Look Better Program, I plan to do the following to continue seeing changes in my physique:

_____

_____

_____

Long-term, I want to see the following changes in my body:

_____

_____

_____

I would like to accomplish these long-term goals by (specify dates, weeks, months, years from now):

_____

_____

Beyond looking better, I want to reap the following benefits from my workouts:

less stress, more energy,
better temper, etc.

When I accomplish all of these goals, I will be:

I will be a new person
& look at things differently

I know these goals are realistic for me because:

Because its what I
& I do it as myself & I can
go well doing performing now
more (xg). ( )

GOAL DIGGER FEEL BETTER LOG:
The last time I felt consistently good was:

What's motivating me now to elevate my energy levels and mood and to feel better overall:

By the end of my first 14-Day Feel Better Program, I want to see the following changes in my energy levels, mood, and/or overall sense of well-being:

_____

_____

_____

After completing my first 14-Day Feel Better Program, I plan to do the following to continue seeing changes in my energy levels, mood, and/or overall well-being:

_____

_____

_____

Long-term, I want to see the following changes in my energy levels, mood, and/or overall well-being:

_____

_____

_____

I would like to accomplish these long-term goals by (specify dates, weeks, months, years from now):

_____

_____

_____

Beyond feeling better, I want to reap the following benefits from my workouts:

_____

_____

_____

_____

When I accomplish all of these goals, I will be:

_____

_____

_____

I know these goals are realistic for me because:

_____

_____

_____

GOAL DIGGER PERFORM BETTER LOG:

The last time I felt I was performing at my peak was:

_____

_____

_____

What's motivating me now to push my performance to its greatest level ever:

_____

_____

_____

By the end of my first 14-Day Perform Better Program, I want to see the following changes in my physical abilities:

_____

_____

_____

After completing my first 14-Day Perform Better Program, I plan to do the following to continue seeing changes in my physical abilities:

_____

_____

Long-term, I want to see the following changes in my physical abilities:

_____

_____

_____

I would like to accomplish these long-term goals by (specify dates, weeks, months, years from now):

_____

_____

_____

Beyond performing better, I want to reap the following benefits from my workouts:

_____

_____

_____

When I accomplish all of these goals, I will be:

_____

_____

_____

I know these goals are realistic for me because:

_____

_____

_____

GOAL DIGGER BETTER HEALTH LOG:

The last time I felt I was my fittest and healthiest was:

_____

_____

_____

What's motivating me now to achieve my healthiest self:

_____

_____

_____

By the end of my first 14-Day Better Health Program, I want to see the following changes in my health and/or physical fitness:

_____

_____

_____

After completing my first 14-Day Better Health Program, I plan to do the following to continue seeing changes in my health and/or physical fitness:

_____

_____

_____

Long-term, I want to see the following changes in my health and/or physical fitness:

_____

_____

_____

I would like to accomplish these long-term goals by (specify dates, weeks, months, years from now):

_____

_____

_____

_____

Beyond improving my health, I want to reap the following benefits from my workouts:

_____

_____

_____

When I accomplish all of these goals, I will be:

_____

_____

_____

I know these goals are realistic for me because:

_____

_____

_____

Appendix 2
Training Journals

As addressed in Chapter 2, it's important to track your progress in your workouts from one day to the next. Doing so will keep you inspired and help you pinpoint how much you're accomplishing. I also recommend that you write down how you're feeling before and after each training session—as well as on the days you don't exercise! I think you'll quickly find you not only achieve everything you're hoping for on the days you train, but your energy levels simply aren't as high if you skip a few days.

< 193 >

Daily**Workout**Log

14-DAY GOAL:

Cardio Workout:

LOCATION	
ACTIVITY	
DURATION	
INTENSITY	
AVERAGE HEART RATE	
DISTANCE (if applicable)	

Strength Workout:

MOVE	WEIGHT (if applicable)	SETS	REPS

What motivated me to work out today:

How I felt before exercising today:

How I felt after completing my workout:

What I learned from today's workout:

SUCCESS JOURNAL

I talked about keeping a success journal in Chapter 5. I suggest making multiple copies of the following sheet and then beginning a daily record of all the things that are going right in your training—and in your life. Read through these entries whenever you hit a motivational snag, and use them to help you recall the passion you had when you first began and to realize how rewarding your fitness quest has been—and can continue to be.

DATE:

The things I did today to further my fitness success ...

MENTALLY:

_____

_____

_____

PHYSICALLY:

_____

_____

_____

NUTRITIONALLY:

_____

_____

_____

OTHER:

_____

_____

_____

_____

_____

_____

The positives that came out of these experiences:

_____

_____

_____

What made these successes particularly gratifying:

_____

_____

_____

Valuable lessons learned from today's successes:

_____

_____

_____

Additional inspiring thoughts about what's possible in my fitness program:

_____

_____

_____

Appendix 3
The Goal Digger Recipes

As noted in Chapter 7, health resorts and spas around the world are encouraging guests to put more time and energy into the meals they cook. These recipes from three of the world's leading destinations—Rancho La Puerta Fitness Resort & Spa in Tecate, Baja California, Mexico; Red Mountain Spa in St. George, Utah; and Lake Austin Spa Resort in Austin, Texas—showcase delicious and nutritious ways to boost your energy, performance, and health, while also helping you manage your weight. Invest some time in the meals you prepare, and take your results to an extraordinary new place.

< **197** >

The**Recipes**: Entrées

Veggie Frittata

1 teaspoon olive oil
½ medium onion, diced
2 cups cauliflower florets
1 small red or yellow bell pepper; or ½ cup carrots, julienned;
   or ¼ cup sun-dried tomatoes
1 cup fresh or frozen peas
3 large egg whites
2 large whole eggs
⅔ cup nonfat ricotta or cottage cheese
2 tablespoons fresh dillweed or chopped basil, or 2 teaspoons dried
Freshly cracked black pepper, to taste
Pinch of ground red pepper (optional)
3 tablespoons grated Asiago or Parmesan cheese

Preheat the oven to 350°F.

Brush a pie plate with some of the oil or coat with cooking spray.

Meanwhile, heat a large skillet brushed with the remaining oil or coated with olive oil spray over medium-low heat. Add the onion; cauliflower; bell pepper, carrots, or tomatoes; and peas and cook, stirring constantly, for 5 minutes, or until tender-crisp. Remove from heat and set aside.

In a small bowl, beat the egg whites and eggs with the ricotta or cottage cheese. Add the dillweed or basil and half of the Asiago or Parmesan. Mix the reserved vegetables into the egg mixture.

Spoon into the pie plate and bake for 20 to 25 minutes, or until eggs are set. Just before serving, sprinkle with the remaining Asagio or Parmesan and return to the oven for several minutes until the cheese melts. Cut into 4 wedges.

Variation: Add 3 ounces of smoked salmon or smoked tempeh such as Fakin' Bacon to the egg and cheese mixture.

MAKES FOUR 7.5-OUNCE SERVINGS

Calories per serving: 166, Carbohydrate: 15 g, Protein: 14 g, Fat: 5 g
(2 g saturated)

—Created by Yvonne Nienstadt of the Culinary Team
of Rancho La Puerta Fitness Resort & Spa

The**Recipes:** Entrées

Turkey Hash Patties with Cranberry Orange Relish

PATTIES
1½ pounds ground turkey, cooked
1 teaspoon ground red pepper
½ teaspoon ground cloves
1 cup apple cider
1 teaspoon hot pepper sauce
1 teaspoon paprika
Pinch of salt
Dash of black pepper

RELISH
6 ounces cranberries
½ orange, including peel
½ tablespoon lemon juice
½ tablespoon fructose

To make the patties: Preheat the oven to 350°F.

In a large bowl, combine the turkey, red pepper, cloves, cider, hot pepper sauce, paprika, salt, and black pepper and mix well. Scoop 1-ounce portions onto a parchment-lined baking sheet, flatten scoops into patties and bake for 8 to 10 minutes.

To make the relish: In a food processor, combine the cranberries, orange with peel, lemon juice, and fructose. Pulse until ground together. Serve at room temperature.

MAKES 8 SERVINGS (1 PATTY + 2 TABLESPOONS RELISH EACH)

Calories per serving: 156, Carbohydrate: 7 g, Protein: 15 g, Fat: 7 g

—Courtesy of Red Mountain Spa, St. George, Utah

Blackened Salmon

¼ **cup paprika**
2 teaspoons onion powder
2 teaspoons garlic powder
½ **teaspoon ground red pepper**
1 teaspoon white pepper
1 teaspoon black pepper
1 teaspoon dried thyme leaves
1 teaspoon dried oregano
2 teaspoons salt (optional)
4 salmon fillets (4 ounces each), skin removed
Lemon wedges and melted butter (optional)

In a medium bowl, combine the paprika, onion powder, garlic powder, red pepper, white pepper, black pepper, thyme, oregano, and salt, if using. Mix thoroughly. Pat the salmon dry with paper towels, then dredge the fillets in the seasonings, coating each piece thoroughly. Spray both sides of each fillet with cooking spray. Grill over hot coals, turning occasionally, for 10 minutes per inch of thickness, or until blackened and cooked through. Serve with a lemon wedge or brush with a little melted light butter, if desired.

MAKES 4 SERVINGS

Calories per serving: 187, Carbohydrate: 4 g, Protein: 22 g, Fat: 9 g

—*Courtesy of* Fresh: Healthy Cooking and Living from Lake Austin Spa Resort

The**Recipes:** Soups, Salads, Sides, and Smoothies

Roasted Tomato Soup

1 teaspoon olive oil
2 pounds plum tomatoes
1 medium onion, diced
2 stalks celery, diced
1 tablespoon fresh thyme or 1 teaspoon dried
Salt and black pepper to taste
2 teaspoons olive oil
3 cups vegetable stock
1 cup frozen peas
12 fresh basil leaves, sliced (optional)

Preheat the oven to 350°F.

Coat a baking pan with one teaspoon of the oil. Bake the tomatoes for 20 to 25 minutes, or until tender.

In a large saucepan, cook the onion and celery over medium-high heat in the remaining oil until the onion is translucent. Add the baked tomatoes, thyme, and salt and pepper. Cover and cook for 5 to 10 minutes.

In a blender or food processor, combine the tomato mixture and the stock. Blend or process until smooth. Return to the saucepan.

Add the peas and cook for 5 minutes more.

Ladle into bowls. Garnish with the basil, if desired.

MAKES 8 SERVINGS

Calories per serving: 65, Carbohydrate: 10 g, Protein: 2.5 g, Fat: 2 g

—Created by chef Jesus Gonzalez of La Cocina Que Canta Culinary Center
at Rancho La Puerta Fitness Resort & Spa

Butternut Squash and Coconut Soup

1 tablespoon roasted peanut oil or sesame oil
2 cloves garlic, minced
2 tablespoons minced fresh gingerroot
2 pounds cubed, seeded, and peeled butternut squash
1 small onion, peeled and chopped
4 cups vegetable stock
1 can (13 ounces) light coconut milk
½ teaspoon powdered turmeric
1 teaspoon Asian chili paste
¾ teaspoon salt
1 teaspoon grated lime zest
Lime wedges, cubed tofu, chopped fresh cilantro, and/or basil for garnish

Heat the peanut oil in a 3-quart saucepan over medium heat. Add the garlic and gingerroot and cook, stirring frequently, for one minute until golden. Add the squash, onion, stock, coconut milk, turmeric, chili paste, salt, and lime zest and mix well. Bring to a simmer and cook approximately 30 minutes, until the squash is very tender. Place in a blender or food processor puree, in batches if necessary. Return the puree to the saucepan and cook over medium heat for approximately 5 minutes or until hot. Serve hot, garnished with lime, tofu, cilantro, and/or basil.

MAKES 8 SERVINGS

Calories per serving: 124, Carbohydrate: 16 g, Protein: 2 g, Fat: 6 g

—*Courtesy of* Fresh: Healthy Cooking and Living from Lake Austin Spa Resort

TheRecipes: Soups, Salads, Sides, and Smoothies

Spinach Salad with Hard-Cooked Egg Whites and Toasted Sunflower Seeds

2½ tablespoons sunflower seeds
1 teaspoon Bragg Liquid Aminos*or low-sodium soy sauce
½ teaspoon paprika
4 cups fresh spinach, washed and dried
4 hard-cooked eggs, whites only, sliced
2 navel oranges, peeled and sliced in rounds
*Available in health food stores

In a small skillet, combine the sunflower seeds, Bragg or soy sauce, and paprika. Toast the seeds over low heat, stirring constantly for about 3 to 4 minutes until lightly browned. Remove from the heat and set aside to cool.

Arrange the spinach on 4 plates. Top with the eggs and sprinkle with the reserved seeds. Garnish with the orange slices.

MAKES 4 SERVINGS

Calories per serving: 94, Carbohydrate: 12 g, Protein: 7 g, Fat: 3 g

> —*Created by chef Jesus Gonzalez of La Cocina Que Canta Culinary Center at Rancho La Puerta Fitness Resort & Spa*

Red Mountain Chicken Salad

6 ounces roasted, diced chicken breast
⅓ cup green apple, finely chopped
¼ cup plus ½ tablespoon plain yogurt
¼ cup finely chopped onion
¼ cup finely chopped celery
¾ teaspoon lemon juice

Mix together the chicken, apple, yogurt, onion, celery, and lemon juice.

MAKES ABOUT 5 SERVINGS (½ CUP EACH)

Calories per serving: 73, Carbohydrate: 3 g, Protein: 11 g, Fat: 2 g

—Courtesy of Red Mountain Spa, St. George, Utah

TheRecipes: Soups, Salads, Sides, and Smoothies

Agave French Fries

1 tablespoon olive oil
2 tablespoons Dijon mustard
2 tablespoons agave syrup
1½ teaspoons onion powder
1½ teaspoons garlic powder
1 teaspoon paprika
2 pounds potatoes, cut into strips (like french fries)
Pinch of salt
Pinch of black pepper

Preheat the oven to 325°F.

In a large bowl, mix together the oil, mustard, syrup, onion powder, garlic powder, and paprika. Add the potatoes and toss. Season with the salt and pepper. Place on a silpats or a baking sheet lined with parchment paper.

Bake for 12 to 16 minutes, or until light brown and tender.

MAKES 8 SERVINGS

Calories per serving: 129, Carbohydrate: 29 g, Protein: 3 g, Fat: 2 g

—Courtesy of Red Mountain Spa, St. George, Utah

Banana Almond Smoothie

2 cups plain nonfat yogurt
2 tablespoons chopped almonds
1 medium ripe banana
1 teaspoon cinnamon
1 tablespoon maple syrup, syrup of agave, or honey (optional)

Place yogurt, almonds, banana, cinnamon, and syrup or honey, if
using, in a blender. Puree until smooth. Pour into 3 glasses.

MAKES 3 SERVINGS

Calories per serving: 152, Carbohydrate: 28 g, Protein: 8 g, Fat: 3 g

—Created by chef Jesus Gonzalez of La Cocina Que Canta Culinary Center
at Rancho La Puerta Fitness Resort & Spa

The**Recipes:** Desserts

Blueberry Cobbler

8 cups fresh or frozen blueberries, thawed
1 cup sugar
3 tablespoons cornstarch
Grated zest and juice of 1 lemon
1 cup flour
½ cup rolled oats
1 teaspoon baking powder
½ teaspoon baking soda
½ teaspoon salt
½ teaspoon ground cinnamon
4 tablespoons light butter, cut into small cubes and chilled
¾ cup buttermilk
Low-fat frozen vanilla yogurt (optional)

Preheat the oven to 375°F.

In a large bowl, combine the blueberries, ⅔ cup of the sugar, cornstarch, and lemon zest and juice. Set aside and let stand for 15 to 20 minutes, stirring occasionally. In another bowl, combine the flour, oats, remaining ⅓ cup sugar, baking powder, baking soda, salt, and cinnamon. Refrigerate for approximately 1–2 hours, or until thoroughly chilled.

Work the butter into the chilled dry ingredients with your hands, pinching the bits between your thumb and fingers until the butter is mostly incorporated. Add the buttermilk and stir just until combined. Coat a 4" × 8" baking dish with cooking spray. Arrange the blueberry mixture in the bottom and top with the dough mixture. Bake for 45 minutes, or until the top is crisp and browned. Serve warm with a scoop of frozen yogurt, if desired.

A variety of other fruit, fresh or frozen, can be successfully substituted for the blueberries. We particularly like apples, peaches, and cherries.

MAKES 10 SERVINGS

Calories per serving: 246, Carbohydrate: 53 g, Protein: 4 g, Fat: 4 g

—*Courtesy of* Fresh: Healthy Cooking and Living from Lake Austin Spa Resort

The**Recipes:** Desserts

Candied Ginger Sorbet

1 cup diced banana
1 cup diced mango
1 cup diced pineapple
2–3 tablespoons minced candied ginger
½ cup fresh orange juice
Mint sprigs or fresh berries (optional)

Place the banana, mango, and pineapple on a baking sheet and freeze for several hours. When solid, remove from the freezer and let stand for 5 minutes.

In a food processor, combine the fruit, ginger, and orange juice. Puree until creamy.

Pour into 6 glasses and garnish each with a sprig of mint and a fresh berry, if desired. Serve immediately.

MAKES 6 SERVINGS

Calories per serving: 78, Carbohydrate: 20 g, Protein: 1 g, Fat: 0.5 g

—Created by chef Jesus Gonzalez of La Cocina Que Canta Culinary Center
at Rancho La Puerta Fitness Resort & Spa

FOR MORE INFORMATION ABOUT THE FEATURED SPAS:

Red Mountain Spa
1275 E. Red Mountain Circle
St. George, UT 84738
435-673-4905
(800) 407-3002 (U.S. and Canada)
www.redmountainspa.com

Lake Austin Spa Resort
1705 S. Quinlan Park Rd.
Austin, TX 78732
512-372-7300
(800) 847-5637 (U.S.)
(800) 338-6651 (Canada)
www.lakeaustin.com

Rancho La Puerta Fitness Resort & Spa
Tecate, Baja California, Mexico
(U.S. Reservations Office and mailing address)
1155 Camino Del Mar #777
Del Mar, California 92014
(800) 443-7565 (U.S.)
www.rancholapuerta.com

< **211** >

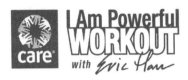

The I Am Powerful Workout with Eric Harr: Call to Action

Inspired by a greater purpose to confront life's hardest challenges head on...

As I finish this book—a work of which I am exceedingly proud—I am taking on another project of which I am exceedingly proud.

I have teamed with CARE, a global humanitarian organization, for the I Am Powerful Workout with Eric Harr. This 2-in-1 challenge motivates people across the United States to create healthier lifestyles for themselves and, in doing so, to also channel their new energy and support into empowering marginalized women to improve the health and well-being of their families.

As obesity rates soar among adults in the U.S., it staggers me to think this could be the first generation in history whose life expectancy will be shorter than their parents. At the same time, women and their families in developing countries are trapped in poverty, struggling every day to simply eat and get healthy. We need a better balance.

I believe it's important to empower people both near and far. At home, we become empowered when we exercise and live healthier. Farther away, in a place like Mozambique, Africa, for example—where a woman's life expectancy is a little over 40 years—we can help empower women to improve their health and well-being and that of their families. I also believe we need to be inspired by a greater purpose to confront life's hardest challenges head on.

That is why CARE and I have come together to launch this campaign. I am training for the Hawaii Ironman Triathlon World Championships in

< 213 >

October in order to raise money and awareness to fight global poverty through CARE. I've asked everyone I know—and some complete strangers!—to donate money on my behalf directly to CARE, and the response has been overwhelming.

Here's what I'm asking you to do: Read this book, challenge yourself, and set an ambitious fitness goal: you know, the one that has been burning inside you. Maybe you want to lose a few pounds, climb a mountain, or train for your first marathon. Get inspired. Get moving. Get your friends and family behind you, and ask them to support you however they can. Maybe they'll give money. Maybe they'll give time. Maybe they'll join you! Then, channel all of your new energy to live your best life—as you help others live theirs.

For more information about this campaign, visit www.care.org/workout to learn the simple steps you can take to get involved. The Web site includes all of the information, fundraising tools, guidance, and support you need to achieve your boldest fitness goals—and to raise money and/or awareness for CARE. You'll have the opportunity to share your own success stories, too.

They say the journey of a thousand miles begins with a single step. So take that first step: Visit the Web site—and know that every step you take toward a better life for yourself will be a step on behalf of marginalized women and girls worldwide.

* 25% of all royalties from the sale of this book will be donated to CARE.

About the Authors

ERIC HARR is CBS's *Weekend Early Edition* fitness correspondent in San Fra-nEric Harr is CBS's *Weekend Early Edition* fitness correspondent in San Francisco and a former *Los Angeles Times* nationally syndicated columnist and syndicated radio host. He is the author of *Triathlon Training in Four Hours a Week*, *Ride Fast*, and *The Portable Personal Trainer*, and the former founding editorial director of the first-ever paperless, interactive consumer magazine: *VIV* (named after his daughter, Vivienne). He is a professional triathlete, ranked number six in the world in his first year, and has competed in 15 countries. He is an international ambassador for CARE, a global humanitarian organization. Eric is training for the Hawaii Ironman World Championships in October to raise money and awareness for CARE—as he calls on Americans to take on their own fitness challenges and join him in the fight against global poverty at www.care.org/workout. Eric hosts weekly CBS radio segments and a new health/fitness podcast: www.harrcast.com. He lives in Fairfax, California, and in Monte Carlo, Monaco, with his wife, Alexandra and their daughter, Vivienne. To learn more, visit www.ericharr.com.

ALEXA JOY SHERMAN is a freelance writer based outside of Los Angeles. A former senior editor for *Shape* magazine, she specializes in health and fitness and has contributed to a number of national consumer publications, including *Women's Health, Natural Health, Shape, Family Circle*, and *O: The Oprah Magazine*. She is also the coauthor of *The Happy Hook-Up: A Single Girl's Guide to Casual Sex*. However, she is no longer a single girl; she shares a home with her husband, Joel; their beautiful son, Jack; and their spastic dog, Sydney. To learn more, visit www.alexajoysherman.com.

< **215** >

Index

Boldface page references indicate photographs.
Underscored references indicate boxed text.

< **217** >

Goal Digger Logs (*cont.*)
   overview, 183
   Perform Better Log, 32, 188–89
   for refining goals, 13, 27, 31, 32, 35
Goal Digger Survey
   questions, 23–25
   retaking, 23, 26
   scoring, 23, 25–26
   section one interpretation, 26–27
   section two interpretation, 30–31
   section three interpretation, 31–32
   section four interpretation, 32–35
Goals for exercising. *See also* Motivation;
      specific goals
   as actions, not outcomes, 22
   feeling better, 27–28
   Goal Digger Logs for refining, 13, 27,
      31, 32, 35
   Goal Digger Survey questions, 23–25
   Goal Digger Survey results, 26–35
   Goal Digger Survey scoring, 23, 25–26
   health, 32–35
   looking better, 26–27
   mission-driven, 21
   motivation increased by, 13
   payoffs exceeding, 25
   performing better, 28–29
   pinpointing specifically, 22–23
   primary, 26
   prioritizing, 23
   realism about, 26–27, 29
   setting short- and long-term, 28
   variety of, 22
Goggles, 16
Gratitude, as motivation, 12
Growth hormone, 100

H

Health. *See also* Aches and pains; Illness;
      Injury
   boosting immunity, 147–53
   as exercise payoff, 2
   14-Day Better Health Program, 74–85
   as goal for exercising, 32–35
   lack of focus as danger to, 113
   medical checkups and tests for, 32
   One-Day Meal Plans for, 177–81
   refining your goals, 35

tracking difficult for, 34–35
   as weak motivation for many, 34–35
HealthAid America, 148–49
Health professionals. *See* Doctors
Heart disease, preventing, 33, 166
Heart rate. *See also* Maximum heart rate
      (MHR) percentage
   deep breathing for reducing, 113
   elevated in morning, 143
Heart rate monitor, 49
Helmets for cycling, 16, 131
Heroes, inspiration from, 124
High blood pressure, preventing, 33
High-efficiency particulate air (HEPA)
      filters, 151
Hot weather precautions, 140
Houseplants, 151–52
Hydrating
   before exercise, 45, 167
   schedule for, 167
   sports drinks for, 168

I

I Am Powerful Workout, 213–14
Illness. *See also* Aches and pains; Injury
   as excuse for not exercising, 10–12
   paying attention to, 129–30
   prevented by exercise, 33–34
   sedentary lifestyle and risk of, 32
   seeing a doctor about, 11, 12, 130
Immune system, strengthening
   being social for, 152–53
   drumming for, 152
   general recommendations for, 147
   importance of, 147
   indoor pollutant reduction for, 149–52
   laughter for, 149
   quitting smoking for, 151
   stress release for, 148–49, 152
Injury. *See also* Aches and pains; Illness
   acute, 145
   caloric need and risk of, 159
   ceasing activity immediately after,
      143
   chronic, 145–46
   confidence shattered by, 120
   cross-training to prevent, 104–5
   diagnosing, 145–47